COACHING - NUTRITION - ACHIEVEMENT

Smart, Sweaty, and Slightly Out of Sync

A Realistic Guide for Endurance Athletes with a Life

© 2025 Darren Gibbons / Smart Performance Coaching

www.smartperformancecoaching.co.uk

First published in the United Kingdom in 2025.

Acknowledgements

To every athlete who has trained through chaos, cursed during threshold reps, or sent a one-word message that simply read "Help" — this book is for you. You're the ones who laced up on tired legs, found twenty minutes when there should've been none, and kept going when plans on paper met life in progress.

To the early risers, the lunch-break warriors, and the evening grinders — the people who've balanced workouts with work meetings, school runs, sore knees, sniffly kids, and laptops that wouldn't shut down — you're the reason this exists. Smart Performance Coaching was built around real lives because of you.

To the athletes who trusted the process, questioned the process, reshaped the process, and stuck with it anyway: thank you. Your honesty sharpened the system. Your notes — the good, the bad, and the "my watch thinks I'm dead" — made these pages better.

To the Smart Performance Coaching team: your belief, brains, and banter carried this from an idea to a book. You kept standards high and the jokes higher. Special thanks to Rachel Trott, our Level 3 Diet & Nutrition Coach, whose no-nonsense guidance has helped countless athletes fuel like adults, not algorithms. Rachel — your calm, clarity, and care show up in every chapter that mentions food.

To the physios, massage therapists, bike fitters, pool staff, run-shop experts, and all the pros who patch people up and send them back out smarter — we notice you. To training partners who waited at the corner, circled back on windy rides, and clapped for ugly last reps — you're part of every finish line.

To the families, friends, and colleagues who carried bags, watched kids, asked real questions, and pretended not to mind the drying rack of lycra — thank you for lending your patience to someone else's goal. To baristas who knew the order, lifeguards who opened the gate two minutes early, and neighbours who didn't complain about turbo noise — you made consistency possible.

To the early SPC athletes who said, "I'll try it your way for a month," and then kept going for seasons — your results and feedback shaped the framework more than any textbook.

And finally, to you — the reader holding this now. Thanks for giving your attention to something that asks for effort, not shortcuts. I hope these pages help you train with more confidence, more control, and a little more enjoyment. If they do, it's because of the people above.

Introduction — Real Life, Real Training

Let's get this out of the way: you don't need to train like a monk, live like a monk, or eat like a monk to be an endurance athlete. You don't need to shave your legs, drink beetroot smoothies that smell like compost, or post sunrise selfies captioned "no excuses." You just need a plan that works in real life — not in a vacuum. One that allows for kids, families, night shifts, weekends, hangovers, lost motivation, and the occasional full-body existential crisis during a long run.

Because let's face it: you probably didn't become an athlete to live a joyless existence. You didn't pick triathlon, marathon, cycling, or swimming because you love spreadsheets or blisters. You picked it because something about endurance spoke to you — that slow burn of progress, that deep satisfaction of earning something through effort, and maybe, just maybe, that quiet rebellion against the version of yourself that used to avoid PE lessons.

Why This Book Exists

There's no shortage of training books out there. Some promise to make you faster. Others promise to make you unbreakable. A few might even suggest you need to give up carbs, sleep in an altitude tent, and start calling your threshold pace your "sacred zone."

This is not one of those books.

Because if you're anything like the athletes I coach, you're not training in a laboratory. You're fitting in a run between work calls. You're negotiating with toddlers to let you foam roll in peace. You're mentally calculating how many gels you can justify buying before your partner questions the grocery bill again.

You're trying to do the thing — to train hard enough to feel proud, but not so hard that you forget why you started.

That's why Smart, Sweaty and Slightly Out of Sync exists. It's about finding the sweet spot — that messy, glorious middle ground between being all-in and all-burnt-out. It's about learning how to build fitness, consistency, and confidence without sacrificing your sanity or your social life.

Real People, Real Training

You picked this up because you're a real human trying to train inside a very real life. You want to get better, but you also want to enjoy it. You've got ambitions, sure — maybe a marathon, a triathlon, a personal best you've been chasing for years. But you've also got a thousand group chats to keep on top of, dodgy knees, and a recovery score that thinks you're clinically dead every time you stay up past 10 p.m.

You want to know if it's still possible to reach your goals when your week includes kids' homework, late-night emails, and that mysterious shoulder pain that appeared after sleeping "funny."

The answer: yes. You can do it — but not by following plans designed for full-time athletes or 25-year-olds with no dependents.

You don't need a physiology degree, a monk's discipline, or a personal chef to make progress. You need balance, belief, and a coach (or system) that gets that life sometimes means missed sessions, surprise deadlines, and pizza nights that run long.

The SPC Philosophy

Smart Performance Coaching was built on one simple truth: the perfect plan is useless if it doesn't fit your life.

Because real performance isn't about chasing perfection — it's about managing imperfection intelligently. The best athletes aren't the ones who train the hardest every day. They're the ones who can adapt when things don't go to plan, who can find a way to keep moving even when the world feels slightly out of sync.

This book will show you how.

It's part science, part storytelling, and part therapy session disguised as endurance coaching. You'll meet athletes who've juggled 5 a.m. sessions with school runs, who've trained through job changes, heartbreaks, hangovers, and heroic buffet performances the night before long rides.

You'll learn the systems, mindsets, and small but powerful habits that separate those who burn out from those who build up. And you'll laugh — hopefully often — because training might be serious, but athletes shouldn't take themselves too seriously.

What You'll Find Inside

Every chapter builds on the idea that performance comes from alignment, not extremism. You'll find practical tools, stories from real athletes, and lessons that apply whether you're chasing a podium or just trying to make it to the start line without injury.

We'll cover:

How to build smarter training plans that flex with your schedule rather than fight against it.

How to recover better (and why "doing nothing" can be the most productive thing you do all week).

How to handle chaos — from sick kids to sudden work trips — without losing momentum.

How to fuel and train without guilt — no magic powders, just honest food and smart timing.

How to use data without losing your mind — because your watch should support your training, not dictate your self-worth.

And yes, there will be some tough love. Because being "Smart" doesn't mean being soft. It means being strategic — about when to push, when to rest, and when to ignore that friend who thinks every run needs to be a race.

A Word on Balance (and Why It's a Myth)

You've probably heard that you need "balance." The mythical idea that there's a perfect ratio of training, family, work, and recovery that will leave you glowing, accomplished, and fully in control.

Let me ruin that myth right now: balance doesn't exist.

What exists is alignment — knowing what matters to you most, and making your training fit that reality. Some weeks will be brilliant. Others will be chaos in Lycra. That's fine. The goal isn't to find balance; it's to stay in motion.

Training isn't a straight line. It's a rhythm — one that constantly changes tempo. Some days you lead, some days you follow, and some days you're just clinging to the beat. The trick is to keep dancing.

If You're Here, You Belong

Maybe you've doubted whether you "belong" in the endurance world. Maybe you scroll through social media and wonder how everyone else looks so composed while you're still learning how to swim in a straight line or clip in without fear.

Let me be clear: you belong here.

This book is for the parent doing intervals in the dark because it's the only quiet hour of the day. For the weekend warrior who trains like a pro until Sunday lunch derails everything. For the beginner who's terrified, curious, and completely hooked after their first 5K.

You don't have to fit a mould. You just have to show up — imperfectly, inconsistently, and fully human.

So, If You're Here To...

- Train hard but not hate your training.

- Stop second-guessing every zone, pace, or plan.

- Become the kind of athlete who enjoys the process, not just the result.

Then welcome to Smart Performance Coaching — where real-world athletes build race-ready results one sensible (and sometimes sweaty) decision at a time.

Grab a coffee. Get comfortable. You've already taken the first smart step.

One Last Thing

All the athlete stories in this book are based on real people — real endurance athletes with real schedules, real setbacks, and questionable opinions about pre-race breakfasts. The lessons are true, but names and identifying details have been changed. Why? Because privacy matters — and because "Dave" sounded better than "The One Who Trained Through Flu and Wondered Why He Bonked."

This book isn't just about training; it's about the humans behind the sessions. It's about learning how to keep moving forward, even when life goes sideways.

Let's begin.

About the Author

Darren Gibbons

Head Coach & Founder, SPC

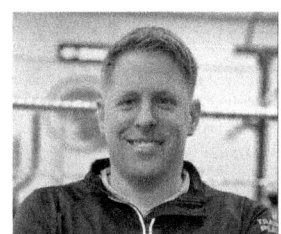

I founded Smart Performance
Coaching for athletes who train in the real world — not a
lab. I coach runners, triathletes and hybrid athletes who
are juggling more than workouts: jobs, deadlines, school
runs, late dinners, and goals that still matter. My approach
is simple: clear structure, flexible execution, and an
athlete-first lens. I use science where it helps, plain
language where it matters, and I care more about your
habits than your watch's mood. Data informs; it doesn't
dictate.

I didn't come to this as an ex-pro. I started as a runner.
Half marathons were my thing because they were simple:
trainers on, out the door, job done. For a long time that
scratched the itch. I chased PBs, collected medals, swore I
was retiring on Sunday afternoon and usually entered
another race on the drive home. After a few years, the
needle stopped moving. I talk a lot in coaching about
"moving the needle"; mine got stuck.

A friend dragged me to a tri club swim. I turned up
expecting a pool full of superheroes and found normal
people doing hard things with a smile. I was hooked — and
suddenly not just a runner, but a terrible swimmer and an

average cyclist. The variety lit me up. I became obsessed with why some athletes thrived while others constantly hit the wall.

I started helping out, took my coaching qualifications, and realised I was more excited about someone else's breakthrough than my own splits. That buzz — seeing an athlete improve because of a cue you gave or a tiny tweak you suggested — is addictive. I never sat down and announced, "Time to build a coaching business." SPC grew out of helping people and wanting to do it properly.

Three years as Chair of Hereford Tri Club taught me plenty — motivation, burnout, and how to herd triathletes who all think they're right. Most importantly, it taught me that training only works when it fits a life. I founded SPC after years of trying to follow plans that ignored reality — the meeting that overran, the poorly child, the long day that ended with an impromptu nap in running kit. There had to be a smarter way to train well without pretending life wasn't happening. So I built one.

When I'm not coaching or writing, I'm fitting in my own sessions, stockpiling Jaffa Cakes, and insisting foam rolling counts as both yoga and life therapy. I'll also politely stop you from doing five threshold sessions in a row "because it felt good."

SPC

Coaching • Nutrition • Achievement — those are the pillars.

SPC isn't "here's a plan, off you go." It's the full picture: how you train, how you fuel, how you recover, and how you keep your head while juggling the rest of life. Our athletes aren't full-time. They're parents, shift workers, small business owners — people spinning plates and still choosing to improve.

The philosophy is simple: train smarter, not harder. That isn't permission to be lazy; it's permission to be purposeful. We don't do grind culture. We do progress without burnout.

"Smarter Than Yesterday" became our north star after years of me comparing myself to everyone else: scrolling, copying, second-guessing. Eventually I stripped it back to what I could control today. One better choice. Pace the session properly. Fuel on time. Sleep. Skip the ego reps. It isn't flashy, but it stacks — and that's the point.

Who We Coach

When I say "athlete", I mean anyone who trains. We coach first-timers and veterans: sprint triathletes, marathoners, Ironman hopefuls, ultra-runners, open-water swimmers. The common thread is real life — jobs, kids, deadlines — and a decision to improve anyway.

The first change when someone joins? Clarity.

Close the tabs.

Ditch the dozen contradictory plans.

Train with intent, not impulse.

How We Coach

Consistency first. Most people overestimate intensity and underestimate repeatability. You don't need hero sessions; you need sessions you can repeat without wrecking yourself. Every workout has a reason — endurance, technique, intensity or recovery. No junk miles. No ego miles.

We coach the real world, not the perfect one. If you've been up all night with a poorly child, the plan changes. If work's brutal, we flex it. The plan works for the person — not the other way round.

Pacing & control matter. Easy is genuinely easy — finish thinking you could do it again. Hard is honest, not heroic.

Long sessions are about durability and fuelling, not proving fitness. On the bike we keep surges in check; in the pool it's rhythm, breath and maintaining shape; on the run we avoid the no-man's-land between easy and purposeful.

Simple rule: repeat what works, fix what doesn't. Train with intent, adjust for real life, and stack small wins until it looks like momentum.

Community & Culture

Belonging matters. Training alone through winter is tough. We built SPC like a club: group rides, online sessions, meet-ups, and a constant stream of chat that's half motivation, half nonsense. Serious training, not-too-serious people — that's the sweet spot. Accountability with humour travels a long way.

What I Believe

Success isn't only PBs or Strava kudos. It's taking your real circumstances, improving them, setting goals and hitting them.

Endurance sport should be open to anyone. Ability doesn't gate access. Training should be fun, balanced and sustainable.

Triathlon and endurance sport should add to life, not take from it.

If that sounds like how you want to train, you're my kind of athlete.

Contents

Chapter 1 – A Smarter Way to Train

5:02am. The kettle clicked. Early, quiet, ordinary. I stood in the kitchen, waiting for coffee and thinking about the day. Work at nine. School run at eight. A ride to fit in somewhere sensible. The watch on the counter offered its usual opinion about recovery. Useful, sometimes. Not gospel.

Every athlete has a story. Some begin with a clear target — first finish line, long-standing PB, proof they're not done yet. Others start in frustration. They've tried the plans, watched the videos, eaten "better," and still feel stuck.

Mine sat between those two. I followed the advice, did the sessions, ticked the boxes, and still felt like progress had slipped out the side door between Tempo Tuesday and a tired Friday shuffle. The gap wasn't effort. The gap was fit. Most plans I used — and later read as a coach — were written for a tidy week that barely exists. In that world nobody misses a session, everyone sleeps well, and there's always time for mobility.

Real athletes live elsewhere. Work lands on the day you'd planned intervals. A child wakes at 4 a.m. Knees complain during the warm-up. The last two kilometres of a long run feel like pulling a tyre. That's the world this book is for.

I didn't need more volume. I needed a way to train that held its shape inside a normal week. Something clear, flexible, and honest. That idea became Smart Performance — not a magic formula, just a practical way to line up training with the life you actually live.

There was a stretch where I treated the plan like law. If it said eight by one kilometre, I did eight by one kilometre, even with a headwind and tight calves. I wore fatigue like a badge. Then I stopped a run halfway, went home, opened a notebook and wrote three columns: what I planned, what happened, what I learned. The pattern was obvious. Weeks where I adapted — moved a session, shortened one, swapped hard for easy — were the weeks I improved. Weeks where I forced it flatlined. It wasn't more that worked. It was smarter.

I started helping a few friends in the same way. We built around fixed points in their week instead of pretending they didn't exist. The plans looked simple. They worked. Word spread. That's how coaching began for me — not with a grand plan, just practical fixes that made sense.

There's a story I come back to often. Let's call him Dave. First 70.3 on the calendar. Three kids. Full-time job. Knees that weren't thrilled about stairs. He downloaded a plan written for someone with free evenings and perfect recovery. Week four: tired, sore, and convinced he wasn't cut out for it.

He wasn't lazy. He was following the wrong plan for his life.

We deleted the second weekly "quality" run. Moved the long ride to a time the house actually allowed it. Added two swing days that could slide without drama. We wrote down clear session purposes so he knew what mattered if time tightened. In a few weeks he went from clinging on to feeling in control. He finished sessions with a little in the tank. Confidence returned. On race day he didn't set records. He finished well, upright, and proud — family there, knees intact. That's the point.

Coach's note: Volume didn't fix Dave's training. Fit did. When training lines up with your week, stress becomes productive instead of punishing.

For years endurance culture has sold "more." More miles, more intensity, more data. And I suppose it works until it doesn't. That takes your recovery and enjoyment with it. Smart training is quieter. It repeats. It fits. It asks a simple question: what's the smart approach I can do this week to move forward? Not the most I can survive.

This isn't about lowering ambition. It's about removing noise so the important work actually happens. If you've ever swapped a junk session for sleep and felt better two days later, you've met the idea already.

One winter I helped a parent of two rebuild after a messy stretch. We started with fixed points: school runs, one reliable evening, one early morning. We built five sessions inside that frame. Nothing longer than ninety minutes. Everything got done. Consistency stacked. Six months later they raced calmer and faster than any previous season. No secrets. Just a plan that matched reality.

Coach's note: A plan that can't bend will break. A plan that bends can last.

This book isn't a textbook. You won't find flowcharts or 47 interval types. You won't need a lab or a chef. You'll get stories, clear ideas, and simple structures that hold up in a normal week. You'll also get permission — to adapt without guilt, and to treat recovery as part of training instead of a bribe.

If your plan expects ninety minutes on a Tuesday with no context, if "Zone 4" is written with no explanation, if the whole thing collapses the moment you move a day, it wasn't written for you. Good training asks why this, why now, why you. It evolves as you do.

Here's the core of how I work and how this book reads. First, clarity: know what each session is for. "Because it's on the plan" isn't enough. Second, structure: put hard where it belongs, and make easy truly easy. Third, adaptability: build flex around the actual moving parts of your week — work, kids, travel. None of that is soft. It's the difference between lasting a month and lasting a season.

You'll see these ideas through different lenses as we go — running, swimming, cycling, strength, season planning, recovery, race day, mindset, data. Not as a lecture. As a conversation with practical edges you can use.

There's a skill that doesn't get much attention: ending well. The last five minutes easy. The choice to stop one rep before form breaks. The decision to fuel earlier than you think. These small things add up faster than one big heroic session done on fumes. I've coached plenty of people who could suffer. The ones who progress learn when not to.

Coach's note: You don't earn fitness by ignoring fatigue. You earn it by giving your body space to adapt to the work you've already done.

If you've read this far, you probably recognise yourself in parts of this. Maybe you've had a season where the plan ran you instead of the other way around. Maybe you've felt the pressure to do more when the sensible answer was different work, or less of it. That's normal. The goal isn't perfection. It's a rhythm you can keep.

So this is the offer: train hard enough to get better, and smart enough to stay in the game. Use training that make sense in your week. Let recovery do its job. Keep the parts that work. Change the parts that don't. Build a season you can actually complete.

There will be early alarms, late evenings, sessions that don't land, days where you need to swap or skip. None of that ruins anything. The only thing that does is pretending you live in a timetable you don't.

Progress isn't loud. It looks like showing up most weeks, doing the work you can do well, and leaving enough in the tank that you want to come back tomorrow. It looks like making peace with the idea that a smaller, consistent plan beats a bigger, broken one.

The kettle will click again tomorrow. Same kitchen. Same watch with its opinion. Same choice. Move in a way that makes sense, or chase the idea that effort only counts when it hurts. One of those paths lasts.

Welcome to a smarter way to train.

Chapter 2 - The Coaching Philosophy That Changes Lives

Spoiler: it's not about perfection. It's about people.

You might expect this chapter to open with testing protocols and colourful charts. Smart Performance Coaching wasn't built on that. It was built on people — on choices made in the quiet gaps between sessions, not just inside them — and on one truth that changes how you train: athletes aren't machines. They're humans with habits, hopes, limits, and calendars that do not care what the plan says.

Smart Performance works because we don't just write plans. We coach humans.

Before there was a system, there was a pattern. I kept meeting athletes who were trying hard and still coming up short — not because they lacked effort, but because the plans they followed ignored reality. The plan would say "ninety minutes Tuesday, tempo Wednesday, test Friday," as if the rest of the week would politely stand aside. It never did. Miss one session and the plan felt broken. Miss two and motivation slid away. By the time Sunday arrived, the athlete was convinced they were the problem.

They weren't the problem. The design was.

That was the start of the philosophy in this book. I stopped asking how to make athletes do more and started asking how to build plans that survive a normal week. Not softer. Smarter. Sessions with a clear purpose. Structure that holds under pressure. Space to adjust without guilt. A way of training you can repeat when life isn't tidy — which is most of the time.

Coach's note: A plan that only works on a perfect week isn't a plan. It's a wish.

How most plans miss the point is simple. They assume compliance. They assume perfect sleep and steady energy. They assume a body that always agrees. Real athletes live somewhere else entirely. The week at work explodes. A child gets ill. A back grumbles after strength. By Thursday you feel behind. By Friday you're negotiating with yourself. Saturday turns into a tidy-looking session done on fumes, followed by two days of feeling worse.

You don't need a lab to predict what happens next: skipped sessions, self-doubt, and the thought that maybe you're not cut out for this. The issue isn't motivation; it's design. If the plan can't flex, it will fracture. When it fractures, confidence goes with it.

Smart Performance begins with different assumptions. Life will interfere. Training must adjust. Mental bandwidth matters as much as fitness. The athlete who keeps showing up imperfectly will always outperform the one who burns bright and disappears.

Every coach has a philosophy, written down or not. Ours is short, practical, and built from years of watching what actually holds up.

Train like a human, not a spreadsheet.

Build identity before intensity.

Clarity beats complexity.

Motivation is unreliable; structure isn't.

Progress starts when you stop chasing perfect.

Those lines are not slogans. They are filters. Everything passes through them: how we plan weeks, how we talk about success, how we respond when things go wrong. The result is training that looks ordinary on paper and works in real life. Repeatable weeks. Pressure where it matters. Enough space to keep moving when life gets loud.

Jo arrived organised and permanently tired. Years of self-coaching had given her consistency and a habit of measuring herself by outcomes. Good race: confidence. Bad race: collapse. One DNS and she questioned if she was "still an athlete."

We stripped it back. The first block didn't aim to sharpen speed. It aimed to steady identity. What does it mean to train like an athlete when no one is watching and nothing is going to social media? We kept the sessions but changed the questions. Did this help you grow? Did you show up when it wasn't convenient? Did you adapt rather than abandon?

Two months later she said, "I train like an athlete now — not someone pretending." The times improved, but only after belief did. That order matters.

Coach's note: Confidence built on behaviour survives a bad result. Confidence built on outcomes does not.

Mark came in with colour-coded spreadsheets, three dashboards, and a resting heart rate he checked like a stock price. He wasn't short on data. He was short on signal. Every run was a test. Every test was a verdict. He had no training days — only exams.

We narrowed the focus. One intent per session, one or two metrics to check, then put the watch down. He learned to end while moving well instead of chasing one more rep to satisfy a graph. He discovered what easy actually felt like and why it matters. Six weeks later he used the word "calm" about training for the first time. The work didn't get easier. It got clearer.

Coach's note: Data helps when it answers a question you actually asked.

Aisha was a comeback. Months off after an injury and a loss of confidence that didn't show up in any file. She could complete the sessions on good days but braced for bad news every time she laced up. The more reassurance she chased from metrics, the tenser she became.

We rebuilt from the ground up. Short sessions done well. Controlled progressions. Regular check-ins that asked about fear as much as fatigue. She learned the difference between discomfort and danger. The big win was not a race. It was the moment she noticed she had stopped flinching.

Coach's note: Coming back isn't about proving you're unbreakable. It's about building enough trust in your process that you move without bracing.

Parents often ask for the "family version" of a plan, as if it is a different sport. It isn't. It is the same sport with honest constraints. One athlete, two kids, shift work, pool access at awkward times. We didn't add hours. We removed non-negotiables. Five sessions a week, nothing longer than ninety minutes, two sessions that could float, one that could be scrapped without guilt. It didn't look impressive. It built the strongest season they'd had.

Smart doesn't win by being big. It wins by being repeatable.

Perfection is a trap. There will be missed sessions, tired weeks, and days where the best choice is getting changed back out of kit. That isn't weakness. That is honesty. Training is not an exam. It is a conversation with your body and your life. Some days that conversation says, "Walk and call it a win."

Smart Performance is not soft. It is sustainable. We still push and test. We just refuse to trade long-term progress for short-term proof. The athletes who learn that difference don't fade. They accumulate seasons.

Coach's note: You don't get fitter by ignoring fatigue. You get fitter by letting your body adapt to the work you've already done.

The part of coaching that matters most does not show in a plan. It shows in what happens between sessions. We ask questions a watch can't: How did that feel? What else is happening this week? Where is your energy going that we didn't account for?

That dialogue changes everything. Athletes begin to see links between sleep and performance, stress and recovery, confidence and consistency. Once they see those links, they stop guessing. They start making better calls, even when no one is there to advise them. That is the goal — not dependence but understanding.

Coach's note: Good coaching makes you less dependent on coaching.

Dan, a paramedic and father of twins, missed more sessions than he completed in his first month. Nights ran long. Days were full. We set new rules: no guilt. Two anchor sessions per week. Anything beyond that was a bonus. Pressure dropped, rhythm appeared, training stopped feeling like a second job. Six months later he finished his first Olympic triathlon upright and still talking. The story was not the event. It was the months that made the event possible.

Consistency is not doing everything. It is doing enough, often.

Here is what holds the philosophy together when life is not tidy.

Clarity is first. Know why you are doing a session. "Because it is on the plan" is not enough. When you can say the purpose out loud, you cut noise.

Structure is next. Put hard work where it belongs. Protect easy days so they are actually easy. Give recovery the same status as training, because it is training.

Adaptability finishes the picture. Life moves. Plans should too. Shuffling a session is not cheating; it is design. The plan that bends is the plan that lasts.

You will see these ideas again — in running, swimming, cycling, strength, season planning, recovery, race preparation, mindset, and data. The shapes change. The foundation does not.

There are quiet skills that rarely get attention and change everything.

Starting honestly. Not with a heroic first rep to prove a point, but with a warm-up that tells you what is there today. You make better choices when you start by looking rather than guessing.

Ending well. The last five minutes easy. The decision to stop one rep before form breaks. The small habit of fuelling earlier than you think. These do not make highlight reels. They make seasons.

Resetting quickly. Bad sessions happen. The skill is not avoiding them; it is not dragging them into the next one. Write the note. Learn the lesson. Move on.

Coach's note: Fewer stories. More decisions. Better seasons.

What does this look like across a week? Not a perfect grid. A frame that fits. One athlete with a standard office schedule, two school runs, and indoor bike access. We anchored a threshold run on Tuesday evening when childcare was reliable, a sweet-spot bike on Thursday morning before work, and a long ride Sunday morning before the house woke up. We left Friday as a swing day: twenty to thirty minutes easy or nothing at all. We didn't chase volume. We chased repeatability. Eight weeks later the fitness tests moved in the right direction and the notes sounded different: less apology, more clarity.

The plan wasn't exciting. It was sustainable.

A lot of people ask what makes Smart Performance different. The short answer is empathy with structure. We do not treat athletes as inputs and outputs. We look at stress that does not show up in files: the way someone writes about a session, the tone of a check-in, the pattern of short nights. We decide how to push or pull based on the person, not just the numbers. That is not guesswork. It is attention.

When you coach like that, athletes don't just get fitter. They get better at coaching themselves. They start to recognise early signs of trouble and early signs of momentum. They learn when to back off and when to press on. That is progress you keep.

If you take only a handful of lines from this chapter, take these.

A good plan fits your life, not just your Strava feed. You are not lazy; you are likely under-supported. Mindset shapes mileage, not the other way around. Smart beats perfect. Every time.

Those are not slogans. They are habits. When you run your training through them, you keep the work that matters and drop the noise.

Pause and apply. Look at the next seven days. Where does your current plan expect perfection? Where can you trade pressure for consistency? What would change if you built confidence inside each session instead of waiting for a race to hand it to you? Write one adjustment. Make it this week. Small corrections compound faster than you think.

This philosophy is not a neat diagram on a whiteboard. It is a daily habit: coach the human, not just the athlete. Meet people where they actually are — in the middle of work, family, fatigue, and ambition. Build systems that hold when life wobbles. Guide athletes through missed sessions and doubt as much as through medals and finish lines.

That is real coaching. That is Smart Performance.

Now that you know how we think, we turn to who you are — the beliefs, habits, and storyline that sit under your training. That map shapes every decision you make.

Next up: The Athlete Identity Map

Chapter 3 – The Athlete Identity Map

You are not your Garmin.

You are not your last race.

You are not today's pace.

Let's start there.

Most athletes don't have a training problem; they have an identity problem. They're trying to train like someone they don't yet believe they are. That gap shows up as inconsistency, self-doubt, and motivation that disappears the moment life gets messy. This chapter isn't philosophy for the sake of it. It's practical. Identity is the frame that makes training stick. When you build identity first, performance follows.

Plans ask what you'll do; identity asks who you'll be while you do it. When identity is vague, a missed session feels like a verdict. When identity is solid, a missed session is just information. Training gets easier the moment your actions and your self-image pull in the same direction. Not because you suddenly love every session, but because you stop bargaining with yourself about whether you're "really" an athlete. You act like one. The doubt fades because the behaviour matches the story. You don't wait for a medal to claim the identity. You practise the identity until the medal is a by-product.

Sara chased outcomes. Sub-2 half marathon. Sub-25 5K. When the number landed, she felt legitimate. When it didn't, the week was a write-off. One missed session and the story spiralled: I'm not consistent. I'm not an athlete. We pulled the numbers out for eight weeks and replaced them with identity goals she could live now: I train four times per week, one can be short. If I'm genuinely fatigued, I back off because recovery is part of performance. After every session, I write two lines: how it felt and what I learned. Nothing dramatic—just behaviours tied to the kind of athlete she chose to be. By week three, her notes sounded different. Less judgement; more observation. By week eight, she was steadier and, not coincidentally, faster. The main change wasn't pace. It was belief.

Coach's note: Your brain resists behaviours that don't match your self-image. Change the image and the behaviour stops feeling like an argument.

Identity answers the quiet question you ask when nobody is watching: Who am I when training collides with life? If your answer only holds when the calendar is clear and you feel fresh, you have a fragile identity. If your answer holds on messy days, you have a useful one. Identity isn't a slogan or a mood. It's a sum of small decisions repeated until they become normal. You don't earn it at the finish line. You practise it every week.

There's a loop we teach because it works: clarity, action, reinforcement, belief. Get clear on the kind of athlete you're becoming—precise and practical enough to live this week. Take one small daily action that matches it; small is the point because small survives real life. Notice it and write it down with plain language—I trained when it wasn't convenient; I cut a rep early to protect form; I chose sleep over scrolling. Repeat that often enough and the behaviour becomes identity. You need less willpower because you're acting in line with who you are. Then you tighten clarity and loop again.

Coach's note: Don't scale actions until they feel automatic at their current size.

Identity is easier to hold when you can see it, so we build from the inside out. Start with values—what must remain intact while you train: family time, health, work standards, honesty. Training that ignores these won't last. Add principles that protect those values, short rules you can remember: Never trade sleep two nights in a row. Easy days are actually easy. Finish with a little in the tank. Turn principles into behaviour you can count: Four sessions per week; one can be twenty minutes. Two-line debrief after sessions—feel plus lesson. Screens off by ten on training nights. Shape your environment so the default path is the easy path: kit laid out the night before, bottles filled after dinner, two "swing" slots that can absorb life. Finally, collect proof. Once a week, review simple evidence without speeches: sessions started on time, nights with seven hours of sleep, times you adapted without binning the day. Put the map somewhere you'll see it. Edit monthly, not daily.

On any day you show up as someone. The overachiever who believes more is always better. The sceptic who half-trusts the plan and tests everything. The exhausted parent squeezing training into gaps. Or the athlete who trains smart, trusts the system, and treats consistency as part of identity rather than a streak. You can be a work-in-progress and still act like an athlete. You can build belief while missing reps. The point is who you decide to be while you train—especially on untidy days.

Coach's note: Identity is most useful on your worst day of the week, not your best.

Two lenses round this out. After months out with an injury, Aisha could do the work physically, but she braced for bad news every time she laced up. We shifted identity from I must prove I'm back to I rebuild well. Proof looked like short sessions done cleanly, controlled progressions, and one weekly check-in about fear as much as fatigue. Her real win wasn't the first race back. It was the month before, when she noticed she'd stopped flinching. She kept a line she could say out loud: I rebuild with patience and precision.

Mark arrived with dashboards and a courtroom mindset. Every run was a verdict. The new identity wasn't I ignore data. It was I use the right data, not all data. We limited each session to one intent and one or two metrics, then put the watch down. He learned to end while moving well, not to feed a chart. His line: I train with signal, not noise.

Language is part of identity. Watch the words. I have to run becomes I run today. I'm behind becomes I'm adjusting. I'm bad at hills becomes I'm learning hills. This isn't pretending; it's accuracy. "Behind" assumes a perfect plan. You don't live in one. "Adjusting" describes what athletes do. Keep one practical sentence for rough days at the door: I'm an athlete. I start small and build. It doesn't have to inspire you. It has to direct you.

Confidence built on outcomes is volatile. Confidence built on behaviour survives. Track behaviour with a simple ledger filled once a week: sessions started on time; nights with seven hours; times you adapted without scrapping the day; instances you fuelled before you faded; one decision you're proud of that doesn't show on Strava. Five lines, no essays. Your brain will forget the wins and fixate on misses. The ledger keeps the record straight.

Coach's note: Confidence grows when you look where it's actually being built.

Identity isn't only willpower; it's design. Reduce friction by staging kit where you'll see it, shoes by the door, a bike ready on the turbo, warm-ups saved as favourites. Protect one evening if mornings are fragile; protect one morning if evenings get hijacked. Make the simplest path the path to movement. Add fuel by planning two snacks that live at work and in the car, deciding the post-session meal before you start, and keeping a bottle on your desk. Fuel is identity: I make it easier to do the right thing. Small decisions compound because that's how mechanics work.

Hard weeks will happen. A useful identity helps you move through them without a story that makes them worse. If you're sleep-deprived, the action is twenty minutes easy or nothing; say, I'm training for the month, not the day. If motivation is low, the action is the smallest start: kit on, five minutes, decide after; say, I start small; I don't negotiate before I begin. If work explodes, defend two anchors and let the rest float; say, I keep the frame and drop the garnish. If a niggle talks, stop the session and swap to something that doesn't poke it; say, I protect the season, not the hour. A plan that survives your worst week is a plan you can trust on your best.

A few traps pretend to be identity. The streak trap turns consistency into fear; the day you should rest becomes the day you "have to move." Switch to anchor consistency—two non-negotiable sessions that define the week. The all-or-nothing trap says if you can't do the full session, you do nothing. Useful identity says you scale, you don't scrap. The "Monday" trap delays the restart to a ritual; useful identity restarts today—scaled, short, simple. The "pro mode" trap copies habits from people with different hours, stress, and support; useful identity builds like you, not like them. Write the one you fall into most, then write the sentence you'll use to counter it.

Identity carries across disciplines but looks specific up close. In the pool: I treat water skills as strength work. You arrive on time, do the drills properly, keep rest honest, and note one cue that worked. On the bike: I build repeatable power. You fuel early, hold steady, finish clean; if the file looks boring, that's good. On the run: I protect easy with discipline. You ignore the watch on recovery days, stay tall late, and stop one rep before form breaks. In strength: I move well before I move heavy. You use full ranges and leave one in the tank. It's not a checklist to memorise. It's a reminder that identity shows up in concrete choices.

Take a normal, imperfect week: office job, school runs, two pool slots, a Sunday morning long-ride window. The sentence for the week might be: I keep the frame and adapt the detail. Anchors are Tuesday threshold run after bedtime, Thursday sweet-spot bike before work, and Sunday long ride early. Floats are one swim (technique plus steady) and one short run or spin that can move or disappear. Proof is simple: anchors completed, one float used, sleep protected once, one adaptation made without apology. If the week goes sideways, the identity doesn't. You kept the frame.

Identity will slip. You'll forget the sentence, skip the ledger, and judge the week by one bad day. Reset quickly. Read last week's ledger. Write today's sentence. Do the smallest action you can do well. Log the two lines after. Move on. No speeches. Athletes with long arcs don't have fewer slips; they reset faster.

Coach's note: Reset speed is a skill. Practise it.

Confidence isn't loud. It's quiet evidence stacked where you can see it. Loud confidence breaks when results don't arrive on schedule. Quiet confidence asks, Did I act like the athlete I say I am? If yes, it grows. If no, it learns. If you need one practice to build it, keep the ledger for eight weeks without missing. Don't make it pretty. Make it true.

You also become the kind of athlete you see often. Choose one or two people whose training reflects the identity you want. Not the fastest—the most stable. Share weekly wins and lessons with them in short, honest notes. No performance theatre. This isn't pressure; it's alignment. You're reminding each other who you're trying to be.

If you take only a few lines from this chapter, take these: you don't become an athlete at the finish line; you become one when you train with intent. Identity fuels consistency. Consistency drives results. Train like the athlete you're becoming, even when it's messy.

Pause & apply: write one sentence that describes your identity for this month; choose three behaviours that prove it this week (make one of them twenty minutes or less); set up your environment tonight so tomorrow's start is easy; start the ledger with five lines, once a week, no essays. Do it for four weeks. Then edit. Identity isn't a tattoo. It's a decision you keep making.

You can have the best plan, the best gear, and the best intentions. If identity and behaviour don't match, the plan won't stick. Build the identity. Reinforce the behaviour. Results follow because you're acting like the person who gets them. This is who I am. This is what I do. Not only on clear-sky days, but on the ordinary days when the schedule doesn't care. That's where transformation lives—small acts of self-respect repeated more often than not. Identity-based training isn't something you do for a result. It's something you do because it reflects who you've decided to be.

Chapter 4 – From Confusion to Clarity

Let'scut through the noise. If you've ever stared at a plan and thought, What's threshold again? Why am I doing this? Should it feel this hard—or am I broken? you're not alone. Most athletes aren't short on motivation. They're short on clarity. Clarity is the difference between ticking off a session and understanding why it matters. It lets you go to bed knowing tomorrow has a purpose—not just because it's "on the plan," but because it moves you forward. Clarity turns effort into progress. It also gives you permission to rest without guilt. When you understand the why, you can trust the work.

Most plans are built on good intentions and bad instructions. You're handed tempo runs, sweet-spot intervals, aerobic volume and race-pace work—without a translation into your body and your context. Or you're told to ride at a percentage of an FTP you never tested, run at a percentage of a max HR you don't know, swim at CSS plus a number that sounds official and isn't. If you don't know what a number means, it isn't coaching. It's guesswork dressed up. The fallout is predictable. Easy days get run too hard. "Threshold" days slide into the red. You panic when pace doesn't match mood or terrain. You feel guilty for backing off and confused about whether you're underperforming or just mis-pacing. All of it is preventable with a simple structure and a bit of translation.

Clarity comes from three pillars. First, every session must have a single purpose, stated in one line. Easy supports recovery and the aerobic engine; it is not a place to show fitness. Threshold is controlled hard you can repeat; it is not collapse. Long work builds durability and calm fuelling; it is not heroics. Fast work is about economy and turnover; it is not a toughness test. Second, use zones you understand. RPE is always available and it teaches feel. Heart rate is useful when sleep, hydration and temperature are steady. Pace and power are excellent when terrain and setups are stable. Your notes—how it felt and what you learned—are the layer that makes the rest useful. Third, build in blocks. Weeks that nudge stress up are followed by planned downshifts you schedule, not "earn," with short calibration checks every four to six weeks. Stop treating every week like an exam. Progress has a rhythm.

Pete was all-or-nothing. Every run felt like a race, every ride like a test, every swim like a benchmark. Two injuries, one DNS, and an expensive weekend spectating later, he asked for help. He didn't need more fitness. He needed gears. We defined each gear by feel and intent. Easy meant easy. Threshold meant controlled hard, even pacing. We treated Zone 3 with respect, fuelled before he faded, and taught him to end sessions while moving well instead of proving a point. Six months later, he was fitter and finally consistent—not because he trained harder, but because he knew why he was doing what he was doing. Coach's note: You're not undertrained if you can't hold Zone 4 while sprinting hills with friends. You're off-plan.

You don't need a dozen labels to use zones well. Keep the language boring and clear across swim, bike and run. Zone 1 is easy: you can talk comfortably, and you finish fresher than you started; it supports recovery, circulation and technique. Zone 2 is comfortable steady: you can talk but not deliver a speech; it's sustainable and perfect for long work, durability and fuelling practice. Zone 3 is the middle ground: honest but sneaky, fatiguing if you live there; use it on purpose for race-specific segments or strong finishes, not as your default. Zone 4 is threshold: strong, steady and repeatable; breathing is firm, rhythm is steady; it raises sustained power/pace and race control. Zone 5 is short hard work with long recoveries; it builds economy, power and speed; visit, don't live there. Two questions before you move: Which zone am I in? What job is it doing for me today?

Clarity shows up in a normal week. Picture office hours, kids, two pool slots, a turbo and a Sunday long-ride window. Monday is rest or twenty to thirty minutes of mobility—absorbing the previous week and setting up the next. Tuesday is a threshold run with a proper warm-up and three or four six-minute blocks at Zone 4, two to three minutes easy between—controlled hard, even pacing, calm breathing. Wednesday goes to the pool—drills for body position and breath, then six to ten steady hundreds—movement quality first, simple aerobic work after. Thursday is bike sweet-spot: three blocks of ten to twelve minutes at high Zone 3/low Zone 4 with four to five minutes easy; big return for moderate time. Friday is a swing day—twenty to forty minutes easy or nothing—flex built in, week protected, streak ignored. Saturday is a light brick—forty-five to sixty minutes steady bike into ten to fifteen minutes easy run—practise transition without frying your legs. Sunday is a long ride—ninety to one-hundred-fifty minutes steady Zone 2—durability, fuelling and calm control. Notice the lack of drama. Notice the presence of reasons.

Before any session, spend two minutes. Say the purpose out loud. Choose two or three cues you'll actually use—relaxed shoulders, smooth cadence, steady breath. Define what will make it a win—an even split, fuelling on time. Decide your exit plan—how you'll scale if today isn't the day: fewer reps, shorter intervals, or stop when form drops. If you know these, you're training. If you don't, you're guessing.

Mid-session, adjust without guilt. If heart rate is high at easy pace, slow down, shorten the session, or switch to walk/run; the job is recovery, not a number. If threshold pace or power won't hold cleanly, cut the interval length, add recovery, or drop one rep; keep the quality, not the fantasy. If form breaks, end the rep, reset, and either finish cleaner or call it—broken form trains bad habits. If life has cooked you, trade the session for twenty minutes easy or a nap; the rest of the week will repay it. Coach's note: Scaling is a training skill, not a failure.

Keep the debrief short. Two lines: one sentence on feel, one on the lesson. Over time, that becomes your private coach. Patterns will show before they bite.

A few confusions show up often. "I don't know my zones." Start from feel and recent sessions; refine over four weeks.

You don't need a lab to begin. "My heart rate is always weird." It's valuable when sleep, hydration and temperature are steady; when they aren't, let RPE lead and use HR as a secondary check. "Pace on hills is depressing." Pace on a gradient lies; use effort, keep cadence and posture, control breathing. "Power drifts indoors vs outdoors." Accept context; cooling and position change the numbers—track like with like. "I feel guilty changing sessions." Put the exit plan in the plan; planned flexibility removes guilt. "Zone 3 shows up everywhere." Give it a job or avoid it; use it on purpose, not by accident.

You don't need to max out monthly. You need enough data to steer. Every four to six weeks, fold in short checks inside normal training: a twenty to thirty minute controlled-hard run at even pacing; two bike efforts of eight to twelve minutes hard with full recovery, take the best; a 400 + 200 swim time trial with steady pacing. Every week, check subjectively: how did Zone 2 feel, did HR drift, are you sleeping? Update zones when feel and data agree more often than not—not after one heroic or terrible day.

Coach's note: One day doesn't rewrite your zones. Trends do.

Clarity also protects you. If easy days drift faster week by week, if you "can't" run easy unless you hide the watch, if threshold sessions become "survive and hope," if you're under-fuelled in anything longer than an hour, if sleep drops under six and a half hours for more than two nights, if small aches get louder each week—act. Pull one hard session, protect sleep for two nights, add a true Zone 1 day. Fitness won't vanish. Consistency will return.

Words help under stress, so use short scripts. On easy days: Today builds tomorrow. For threshold: Controlled, repeatable, even. For long: Steady, fuel early, finish clean. For bricks: Calm off the bike. On bad days: Scale, don't scrap. On travel weeks: Keep the frame, drop the garnish. These aren't slogans. They're instructions you can follow when you're tired.

Across disciplines, clarity looks specific. In the pool, choose one technical cue per set—long exhale, hips up—and descend effort across the work rather than chasing random speed; keep rest honest and finish with a hundred or two easy to lock the feel. On the bike, set cadence, a fuelling plan, and one posture cue; indoors, fan and bottle in place before pedals; outdoors, match terrain to session. On the run, make the first kilometre slow on purpose, stay tall when tired, keep strides relaxed not frantic; if heart rate drifts ten beats at the same pace on a warm day, you're not failing—you need water and shade. In strength, move well before you move more; when form drops, load drops; two compound lifts done well beat seven done carelessly.

Plans should survive real life in three versions. Plan A is as written: threshold run Tuesday, sweet-spot bike Thursday, long ride Sunday, plus swim, brick and a swing day. Plan B is when work explodes: keep the threshold run, turn Thursday into forty minutes Zone 2, trim thirty minutes from Sunday, slide the swim to the swing day, skip the brick; purpose preserved, stress reduced. Plan C is when sleep collapses: Tuesday becomes thirty minutes easy, Thursday keeps the bike but with one fewer rep, Sunday becomes seventy-five minutes steady with fuelling focus, and you add one nap; confidence preserved, momentum maintained. Clarity is why all three count as progress.

Fuelling is the quiet part of clarity. If a session is longer than sixty to seventy-five minutes, plan it. Simple carbs and fluid beforehand, regular sips during, carbs earlier than you think on the bike, protein and carbs within an hour after. Write it into the session notes. "Fuel early" is a cue, not a vibe.

When athletes say they finally trust their training, they mean they know what they're doing and why. That's clarity.

It shrinks the gap between plan and practice. It makes it easier to start, adjust and end well. Confidence isn't a feeling you wait for; it's a result of clear actions repeated often.

If you take only a few lines from this chapter, take these: clarity beats effort; you don't need to train harder, you need to train on purpose. Every session has a job—know it and respect it. Training too hard too often isn't brave; it's burnout in disguise.

Pause & apply: before your next session, write one line of purpose and one cue; after it, write two lines—feel plus lesson. Look at your week and replace one guess with a clear instruction. Add one swing slot and use it without apology. Do that for two weeks. Notice how much lighter training feels when you know why you're doing it.

The rest of this book will give you the tools, templates and sessions we use at Smart Performance Coaching—but none of it matters without clarity. Get clear first. The work gets simpler. The results get steadier. And training starts to feel like it fits.

Chapter 5 – Swimming: Mechanics, Breathing & Race Prep

Swimming spooks more athletes than the other two disciplines put together. For triathletes it's the leg that can hijack a whole day. For runners crossing over, it's humbling. For time-pressed adults, it's a timetable: lanes, closures, forgotten goggles, and a cap that never wants to cooperate. The aim here isn't a perfect stroke. It's a repeatable one. You don't need elegance; you need efficiency you can hold, breathing you can control, and enough composure that open water feels like a place you know, not a place you survive. That's the lens for everything that follows: mechanics first, then breathing, then load, then race prep. Put those pieces in that order and the water stops arguing.

Most adult swimmers struggle for the same reasons. Body position drifts, hips sink, the head pops up to "find air," which sinks the hips further. Rotation is either flat (all shoulders) or excessive (you snake down the lane). Breathing gets held too long, CO_2 climbs, panic hums, the next breath is snatched, the head lifts again, the rhythm breaks again. Timing is off so the pull presses water down instead of back, and the shoulders do everything. Add a busy lane and a wetsuit and you get tight traps, short strokes, and a rising heart rate that has nothing to do with fitness. The instinct is to push harder. The fix is the opposite. Skills first, then volume. Short sets that wire the pattern, then simple swimming that holds that pattern. If a set gets messier the longer it goes, you don't need more metres; you need better mechanics. Coach's note: choose one focus per length. One cue held well beats five cues held badly.

Start with body line. Head neutral, eyes down or slightly forward, neck long, ribs tucked. You're not trying to "glide." You're trying to travel without wobble. Rotation comes from the trunk, not just the shoulders. About 30–45° each side is plenty: flat and you can't set a catch; over-rotated and you lose stability. A steady two-beat kick is enough for most triathletes; it's timing, not power: left kick pairs with right hand catch, right kick pairs with left hand catch. Catch early, make the forearm vertical, elbow stays high, press water back rather than down. Keep the path close to the body, exit by the hip, recover with a relaxed elbow and quiet hand. Recovery is the easiest place to waste energy; if it's tense, everything else will be.

Breathing sits across all of that. Almost every "I can't breathe" problem is a CO_2 problem and a head position problem. Exhale in the water — slow bubbles, all the way. Turn to breathe; don't lift. One goggle in, one out is a decent guide. Use a simple pattern that keeps you calm: every two on your settled side in chop, every three in a quiet pool if symmetry helps you relax. Own a reset breath: one long exhale, one calm inhale, then back to rhythm. If breathing feels frantic, shorten the repeat, slow the tempo, and rebuild the exhale. Don't add effort. Fix the air first.

Now add load. Only once you can hold the shape under light stress do you layer volume, intervals, and race-specific skills. It's not an anti-fitness stance; it's sequence. Wire the movement, then stress the movement. That sequence saves shoulders and time.

Drills have a job here, but only a few earn their place. Sculling teaches pressure on the water and the feel of an early vertical forearm. 6/3/6 and 3/3/3 (kicks on one side, roll, repeat) build balance, timing, and calm breath. Fingertip drag or a brief pause at entry cleans recovery and hand path. "Polo" (short sets with eyes forward) strengthens posture and sighting without losing the hips. Small pull sets with a buoy (and light paddles if your shoulder is happy) isolate the path and teach you to push straight back. Breathing ladders — two, three, two, three — build rhythm under rising effort. The pattern is always the same: 25–50 m of drill, then swim with the same cue while it's fresh. If a drill doesn't transfer to your stroke within a length or two, it's a distraction. And keep the equipment simple. A buoy, small paddles, short fins, maybe a snorkel and a tempo trainer if they help you feel pace. No gimmicks, no bulging mesh bag. Two tools used precisely will beat ten used randomly.

Open-water composure is a separate skill. You can be fine in a pool and unravel the moment your face meets brown water. The fix begins before you swim. Three long exhales at the shore. Suit pulled properly into the armpits and hips so it doesn't choke your shoulders. A sighting plan you already practised in the pool. The first minute calmer than you think. Breathe every two if you need it. Find feet you can sit on without tapping them. If you get boxed in, soften the hands, angle to open water, settle, and then re-enter the line. Sight just enough to hold your course; if you're on feet and calm, you can sight less often than you think. Wetsuits deserve a line of their own. If the suit isn't high enough, it will round your shoulders and shorten your stroke. Pull from the ankles and wrists upwards in little shuffles until the crotch and armpits are truly high. That one minute of faff saves you twenty minutes of fighting.

Practice on and off, and practice getting out of it: zip, sleeve peel with cap inside, heel pop. You'll thank yourself when your hands don't feel like claws in T1. Coach's note: open water rewards composure more than fitness. Calm first, then speed.

Lucy's story is the right example. She could swim. Open water was the problem. First hundred metres and the world closed in: rushed breath, tight chest, exit to kayak. We changed the target from pace to composure. On land: side-lying kicks with long exhale and quick inhale to teach her brain that air was always available. In the pool: sighting every sixth stroke, short "fast-to-calm" segments (a few strong strokes into a deliberate settle), drafting practice with a friend's feet without tapping. In open water: starts wide, first minute calmer than she thought, one cue on repeat — long exhale. Three months later she swam her fastest wetsuit 1,500 m not because she was suddenly fitter, but because she could down-shift when the adrenaline hit.

Race prep is rehearsal, not hope. Put short swims before bikes in training so you know how breathing behaves under time pressure. Practise starts as 50 m "fast-to-calm": twenty strokes strong, settle to steady, sight as you settle.

Learn to draft without tapping. Practise turning buoys by widening a fraction, shortening the stroke for three to five strokes, then lengthening again. Build one or two "confidence sets" that mirror race intensity in open water so your body recognises the feeling on the day. Keep two cue words you can actually hear in your head when it gets noisy: long exhale, quiet hands, find feet — choose your own, but keep them simple.

The week-to-week structure stays plain. One mechanics-first session where drills feed immediately into short swims. One controlled-hard set where you focus on even pacing and clean water pressure. One longer swim where you practise breath, sighting, and calm. If life is busy, make the third session optional or fold elements into a brick: five minutes of band work and three short "settle" reps before you ride are better than pretending you'll fit another hour in a pool you can't reach. And always add a five-minute dryland warm-up: band Y-T-W, scapular push-ups, a few light single-arm pulls along your catch path, and two slow long exhales. It wakes the pattern without tiring the muscles. It's also the easiest win on any swim day.

Here's a simple, steady, repeatable week example.
Monday — Mechanics & Rhythm (45–60 min) 300

easy as 50 swim / 25 drill. 4 × (25 front scull + 25 swim), short rests. 6 × 50 as 6/3/6 (kick on one side, roll, repeat) → flow straight into 6 × 50 swim carrying the same cue. 8–12 × 50 steady (rests just long enough to keep form). 200 easy down. Aim: balance, timing, clean pressure. Win line: one cue held from first 50 to last.

Tuesday — Short Aerobic + Drill Transfer (30–40 min) 200 easy, choice of 2 drills you need (e.g., fingertip drag, catch-up) × 4 × 25 each → 4 × 50 swim "same cue." 8 × 50 @ easy–steady (10–15 s rest), breathe every 3–5 to stay calm. 100 easy down. Aim: make drills show up in normal swimming. Win line: fewer strokes per length or same SPL at easier effort.

Wednesday — Controlled Hard ("CSS feel") (45–60 min) 300 easy, 4 × 50 build. 5 × 200 at controlled hard, 20–30 s rest. (If this frays, do 8–10 × 100 with 15–20 s rest.) 4 × 50 easy–fast–easy–fast. 200 easy. Aim: steady power without rushing; breathing that stays organised. Win line: last rep looks like the first.

Thursday — Recovery Skills / Pull Focus (30–40 min) 200 easy (snorkel if you like). 6 × 50 pull (buoy only) smooth catch, 10–15 s rest. 6 × 50 choice: sight every 6–8 strokes (eyes lift, hips don't). 100 back or easy kick, long exhale. Aim: circulation + feel; zero shoulder stress. Win line: you get out looser than you got in.

Friday — Dryland Strength + Optional Easy Dip (20–35 min) Dryland (no pool required, 12–20 min): band Y–T–W (2×8), scapula push-ups (2×8), single-arm band pull (2×10/side), dead bug (2×6/side), side plank (2×20–30 s/side), farmer carry (2×20–30 m). Optional 10–15 min easy swim with long exhale if you want to loosen up. Aim: shoulder health, trunk stability, stroke path. Win line: feel primed, not sore.

Saturday — Endurance with Skills (40–60 min) Pool option: 300 easy → 3 × (400 steady + 4 × 50 sight every 6) short rest → 200 easy. Open-water option: 5–10 min settle (breathe every 2 if anxious) → 3–4 × 3–5 min firm with sighting, 1–2 min very easy between → 3–5 min calm finish. Aim: durability, sighting rhythm, calm under mild pressure. Win line: finish calmer than you started.

Sunday — Choice: Open-Water Confidence or True Recovery (20–40 min) Option A: Easy OWS loop, stay close to shore; practise "fast-to-calm" starts (20–30 strong strokes → settle). Option B: 600–1000 continuous easy pool swim, breathe pattern steady, count strokes on 4 random lengths. Option C: Full rest if you need it. Aim: bank confidence or bank freshness. Win line: you're more ready for Monday, not more tired.

If the week gets squeezed

Two sessions only: blend Monday's mechanics into Wednesday (drills → short swims → 8–10 × 100 steady/firm), keep Saturday endurance/skills.

Three sessions: Monday, Wednesday, Saturday. Keep Friday dryland (short).

Swim→Bike brick idea: after Wed or Sat, quick change + 20–30 min very easy spin (smooth cadence, long exhale) so horizontal→seated feels ordinary.

Progress (every 4–6 weeks, only if last reps look like first): Add one repeat (e.g., 5 × 200 → 6 × 200) or trim rest by ~5 s. In endurance sets, extend one 400 to 500. Then take a lighter week: keep Monday, reduce Wednesday volume by ~25%, make Saturday mostly calm skills.

Fuel note: show up fed for technique. For anything hard or >60–75 min, take a small carb beforehand, sip during, and eat protein+carb within 60–90 min after. Finish clean.

Progress every 4–6 weeks only when the last reps look like the first: add a repeat (5 × 200 → 6 × 200), or trim five seconds of rest, not both. In the endurance set, extend one 400 to a 500. Then take a lighter week where you keep Monday's session, drop Wednesday's volume by a quarter, and make Saturday mostly calm skills.

Three ways to keep it alive when life gets noisy: Plan A (as drawn): Monday mechanics, Wednesday controlled hard, Saturday endurance/OW. Done. Plan B (work explodes): keep Monday, turn Wednesday into 10 × 100 steady with generous rest, make Saturday 30–45 minutes easy with 8 × 50 sighting. Skills kept, stress down. Plan C (sleep collapses): Monday becomes 25–35 minutes of drills and easy swimming, Wednesday becomes 6 × 100 steady, Saturday becomes 20–30 minutes calm open water with three short fast-to-calm efforts. Habit intact, load reduced.

Tiny tools that help: write one sentence of purpose on your watch — mechanics → rhythm, controlled hard, even, or end steady, sighting. Set a single reminder for sighting in pool skills sets if you like; otherwise count strokes. After each session, two lines only: feel + lesson. No novels. Fuel the week so technique doesn't turn into bonk practice: arrive fed for short technique work; for anything hard or over an hour, take small carbs beforehand, sip regularly, and eat after — protein plus carbs within the hour, then normal meals.

Clarity is what makes all of this stick. One purpose per session. One cue you actually use. One simple breath plan. One exit plan if form breaks. If the plan says "CSS," translate it to controlled hard, even pacing. If the lane is chaos, drop the send-off and swim on rest. If you can't keep technique, shorten the rep and keep the quality. Scaling is not failure; it's how you keep the good work good.

A few common problems show up again and again. Sinking legs? Press the chest slightly forward, eyes down, keep the kick small and from the hips, exhale in the water. Crossing over? Enter in line with the shoulder, think "train tracks," feel the catch under your forearm, not across your body. Shoulder ache? Lose the big paddles, shorten the set, check that the forearm is vertical before you press; add a little scapular work after. Gasping? Longer exhale, shorter inhale, and a calmer first fifty; don't hold your breath to "brace." Pace falling apart? Reduce the length of the repeat, increase rest briefly, insist on clean strokes. When in doubt, make it easier and do it better.

Fuel matters more than most swimmers want to admit. Anything over an hour deserves a plan: a little carbohydrate beforehand, regular sips during, and protein plus carbs within an hour after. If your goal is technique, don't arrive hypoglycaemic and shaky; you'll rush and tighten and call it "focus."

Strength supports this without taking your week hostage. Two short sessions or one done well are enough: band Y-T-

W for the shoulder blades, serratus wall slides, single-arm rows and pulldowns that mimic your pull path, dead bugs and side planks for rotational control, light external rotations for shoulder care, and farmer carries for posture. Leave one in the tank. You're strengthening patterns, not chasing max numbers.

The sets themselves can stay boring. That's good. Boring is repeatable. A clean mechanics session might be 300 easy as 50 swim/25 drill, 4 × (25 front scull + 25 swim) with ten seconds rest, then 8–12 × 50 steady with your cue and fifteen to twenty seconds rest, 200 easy down. A threshold day might be 300 easy, four × 50 building effort, then five × 200 at controlled hard with twenty to thirty seconds rest, finish with four × 50 easy-fast-easy-fast, 200 easy. A pool-based open-water skills set could be 300 easy, then three rounds of (four × 50 sight every six strokes + 100 steady), finishing with six × 50 "fast-to-calm." Four weeks later you can add a repeat or trim the rest. That's progression.

What about weeks that go sideways? Keep the frame. If work explodes, defend one mechanics session and one controlled-hard set; let the third float. If sleep collapses, trade the hard set for twenty to thirty minutes of easy technique work and keep the long swim calmer with sighting practice; catch up on sleep twice. If you feel a shoulder niggle, drop paddles, shorten reps, end while form is clean.

Coach's note: your swim improves most on the days you don't overreach.

Confidence in the water comes from clarity. When athletes say they're finally "okay" in the swim, they usually mean they know what to pay attention to and what to ignore. One cue. One breath pattern. One simple purpose. Decisions shrink; anxiety follows. Calm isn't a mood you wait for — it's a habit you practise.

If you only carry a few lines out of this chapter, take these: don't train your flaws, train your form. Breathing is a skill — practise it like one. Confidence comes from rhythm, not mileage. Visit hard; live at controlled. Technique first. Then rhythm. Then pace.

Pause and apply it now. Choose the cue you'll use next session. Pick the mechanic you'll hold for 8–12 × 50. If form breaks, shorten the rep. Add a five-minute band warm-up before every swim for the next two weeks. Small hinges; big doors.

You don't need the "best" stroke. You need a stroke you can repeat under pressure. Get efficient. Breathe with control. Practise being calm when others aren't. Do that often enough and you'll get out of the water ready — not just relieved, but primed for the bike and everything that follows.

Chapter 6 – Cycling: Strength, Efficiency & Bricks That Don't Break You

Cycling is the glue in triathlon. It's the longest leg, the most kit to manage, and the easiest place to leak minutes you'll never get back. Strong cycling isn't living in aero like you're prepping for Kona, refreshing FTP charts for reassurance, or chasing every KOM you see. Good cycling is strategic, sustainable, and smart. It's riding strong enough to hold pace — and still having legs to run. It's using gears, fuelling, and focus, not just quads. Get the bike right and the rest of the day gets simpler. Get it wrong and the run turns into a long, sweaty lecture in pacing. The aim here isn't a magic number. It's an approach you can repeat. You build an engine you can rely on and a way of riding that protects it. That means strength you can feel in your posture, power you can hold without bargaining, and habits that stay with you when the course, the group, or your own enthusiasm tries to pull you off plan.

Most athletes make the same mistakes. They surge up every rise because it feels brave. They coast little descents because it feels like a break. They eat late because the first hour feels fine. They sit too low when they're tired, jam their hip flexors, and wonder why the last third feels like riding with the brakes on. Then they try to run. The fix isn't heroic. It's sequence and clarity. First, build strength on the bike. Low-cadence work and controlled climbing teach you to push without wobble. Strength here isn't gym numbers; it's posture that doesn't leak power. Second, raise sustainable power with sweet-spot and sub-threshold work — most of the gains for a manageable cost. Third, train transfer: bricks that normalise running off the bike, long rides that rehearse fuelling and patience, and mental skills that keep you steady when the day is noisy. Do those in that order, and you'll arrive at T2 with legs that still feel like yours. Coach's note: If the best five minutes of your week live in the middle of your long ride, you're off script.

Indoors or outdoors? Both — used on purpose. Indoors gives you control and efficiency. You hit the target, manage rest, and keep the heat honest with a fan and bottle. It's ideal for quality when time is tight. Outdoors gives you handling, patience, and terrain decisions you can't learn on a trainer. You discover what wind does to effort, how corners carry speed, and where pacing goes to die on rolling roads. Sharpen inside. Reinforce outside. Match route to session. Even intervals belong on even stretches, not traffic lights and roundabouts.

Bricks need the same thought. They're not punishment. They're transfer sessions. The goal is making the bike-to-run shift ordinary, not epic. Sometimes that means trimming the bike so the run can be done as intended. Sometimes it means doing part of the run on the bike — locking cadence and breath at what you'll use in the first kilometre so the step off the pedals feels familiar rather than chaotic.

Will needed that lesson. Strong cyclist, cooked runner. Every brick ended in a shuffle; every race looked fine until T2. We dialled down bike intensity on key weeks, and on the bike we rehearsed the first two minutes of the run: quiet hands, steady cadence, long exhale. He didn't ride slower. He rode steadier. Off-bike pace dropped by chunks because he arrived with legs — and a plan.

Posture is the quiet win. Fit matters, but posture under fatigue is where time goes missing. A stable rider wastes less energy. Less sway, more speed. What does stable look like? Elbows soft. Shoulders relaxed. Head still. Hips quiet. On climbs, sit tall and keep your pelvis level; don't hinge so far forward you pinch your hip flexors. In aero, think "long from crown to tailbone," not "folded in half." If your shoulders are doing your legs' work, you'll feel it on the run. Seated climbing drills help here: steady torque without rocking, breathe low, keep your sit bones even. Single-leg pedalling smooths the dead spot and shows you where you stomp. Late-session core cues matter most; anyone can look tidy in the first twenty minutes. Hold your shape in the last twenty and your run won't pay the bill. Coach's note: The fastest position is the one you can keep while you breathe and eat.

Fuel is the other quiet win. Most "fade" is fuelling or pacing. Decide before you roll: what, when, how much. On anything over 60–75 minutes, take fluids and carbs early and keep them coming. Indoors, use a real fan and drink more than you think — heat will lie to you about effort. Outdoors, let conditions inform choices: sip regularly in heat, use tailwinds or smooth sections to eat, and accept that higher temperature drives heart rate at the same power. If you "forget" to fuel whenever the pace is good, put reminders on your head unit. Tidy riders eat early. Messy riders chase a hole later.

Pacing stays simple when you let it. Climbing isn't a chance to prove a point; it's a chance to keep your shape. Shift early, not as a last gasp. Keep cadences alive rather than grinding to feel tough. On flats, hold steady and keep the head still. In wind, posture first, ego last. Race day is not a series of surges to win arguments with hills. It's a long conversation with your effort that ends with running well.

Use gears like tools, not trophies. Most age-groupers wait too long to shift, grind up, coast down, and burn matches they won't get back. Smooth is fast. Keep a cadence range that keeps you out of trouble — say 85–95 on flats, 70–85 on controlled climbs unless you're deliberately training low. When the grade bites, downshift early. When it releases, bring cadence up and carry speed, not RPM alone. On descents, free speed is still speed. Light pressure on the pedals, clean line, eyes through the exit. Brake before the corner, not in it. The fastest kilometre is often the one you didn't interrupt. Coach's note: Boring files win races.

Here's a cycling week that actually works — the same clean rhythm you saw in the swim chapter: simple, repeatable, adaptable.

Monday — Recovery Spin + Mobility (20–40 min + 10–15 min) Spin Z1–low Z2 on easy terrain or trainer (high cadence, light pressure). Then 10–15 min mobility: hip openers, thoracic rotations, calves, hip flexors. Aim:

circulation and tissue freshness. Win line: you get off the bike looser than you got on.

Tuesday — Sweet Spot (60–75 min) Warm-up 10–15 min (include 2–3 × 20 s high-cadence spin-ups). Main set: 3 × 12 min @ high Z3/low Z4 (≈88–92% FTP) with 5 min easy between. Cool 10 min easy. Aim: sustainable power without drama. Win line: last block equals the first within a few watts/seconds.

Wednesday — Aerobic Endurance + Posture (60–90 min) Steady Z2 throughout. Every 10 min: 60–90 s "focus window" in aero (or hoods) → soft elbows, still head, quiet hips. Optional 4 × 5 min single-leg emphasis (left/right focus, both feet clipped in) inside Z2 to smooth the dead spot. Aim: durable engine + holdable position. Win line: posture stays tidy in the final 20 min.

Thursday — Cadence & Form (45–60 min) Warm-up 10 min. Main set: 4 × 6 min low cadence (55–65 rpm) @ Z3, 3 min easy between → then 6 × 30 s high-cadence spin-ups (100–110+ rpm), 30 s easy. Cool 8–10 min. Aim: leg strength and neuromuscular snap without frying you. Win line: hips stay quiet at low cadence; spin-ups feel quick, not frantic.

Friday — Strength Support + Opener (20–30 min + 20–30 min) Gym (or home): hinge (RDL) 2–3 × 6–8, split squat 2–3 × 6–8/side, row or pulldown 2–3 × 8–10, suitcase/farmer carry 2 × 20–30 m. Leave 1 rep in the tank. Optional bike opener: 20–30 min Z1–Z2 with 3 × 10 s smooth standing surges. Aim: scaffolding for posture at hour three. Win line: you feel primed, not sore.

Saturday — Long Ride + Short Brick (90–180 min + 10–15 min run) Mostly Z2. Include 1–2 × 20–30 min at top Z2/low Z3 on steady terrain. Fuel early and on schedule. Brick: 10–15 min very easy run (calm feet, long exhale). Aim: durability, nutrition practice, relaxed step into the run. Win line: you finish the run feeling like you could keep going.

Sunday — Recovery Spin or Cross-Train (30–45 min) Z1–low Z2 spin or walk, easy trail jog, mobility/yoga. Aim: circulation, not fitness. Win line: you feel better after than before.

If the week gets squeezed

Two rides only: blend Tuesday + Thursday (10–15 min cadence/form primers → 2 × 12 min sweet spot) and keep Saturday's long ride + easy brick.

Three rides: Tuesday (SS), Thursday (form), Saturday (long + brick). Keep Friday strength short (20–25 min).

Travel week: defend one quality (SS or cadence/form) and one long steady; everything else floats.

Progress (every 4–6 weeks, only if last reps look like first)

Add a rep (3 × 12 → 4 × 10), or trim rest by ~1 min — not both.

In the long ride, extend one steady block by 5–10 min.

Then take a lighter week: keep Tuesday, reduce Thursday volume ~25%, shorten Saturday and keep the brick very easy.

Fuel & setup notes

Indoors: big fan, bottles in reach, towel ready; same trainer calibration each time.

Fuel: >60–75 min? Start carbs early (aim 30–60 g/hr) + electrolytes; eat within 60–90 min after (protein + carbs).

Pacing mantra: Shift early, sit still, breathe low.

Aero rule: fastest position = one you can hold while you breathe and eat.

Coach's note: The session that protects the week is better than the perfect one that cancels it. Finish clean.

Three ways to keep the plan alive when life gets noisy: Plan A (as drawn): Tuesday sweet spot, Thursday cadence & form, Saturday long + brick, Sunday recovery. Done. Plan B (work explodes): keep Tuesday, turn Thursday into 40 minutes Zone 2 with 6 × 30 second spin-ups, trim

Saturday by 30 minutes and keep fuelling on schedule; brick becomes 8 minutes. Plan C (sleep collapses): Tuesday becomes 30 minutes easy with 4 short spin-ups, Thursday becomes 2 × 8 minutes sweet spot if you're fresh (else Zone 2), Saturday becomes 75 minutes steady + 8 minutes very easy run; Sunday off. Habit intact, load reduced. Coach's note: The session that protects the week is better than the perfect one that cancels it.

You don't have to love numbers to use them. One intent per session. One or two metrics you trust. Then ride. RPE never runs out of battery. Heart rate helps when sleep, hydration, and temperature are steady. Power is honest when the setup is consistent. If you like TSS and IF, keep them in the background; they summarise after the fact, they don't tell you how to ride today. Your notes make the data useful. Two lines after the session — feel + lesson — will teach you more than another decimal place. Examples: Felt flat early; came good after 20 — add longer warm-up on SS days. Cadence died on last SE rep — shift sooner. Ran off the bike calmly — first km deliberately slow worked. Coach's note: The best session is the one you can repeat next week.

Common problems, simple fixes. Grinding climbs because "it feels strong"? Shift sooner. Keep cadence alive. Save your quads for the run. Coasting every little descent? Keep light pressure on the pedals in a small gear. Free speed matters. Turning every group ride into a race? Keep one for fun; make the rest serve the plan. Treating aero like a dare? Hold the fastest position you can breathe and eat in for the time you need — then train that. Forgetting to fuel when the numbers look good? Use alarms until it's a habit. Over-braking in corners? Brake before, eyes through the exit, soft hands, stable torso. Confidence grows with repetition. If you always "blow up" at the same point, it's rarely grit. It's a first hour too hot, a second under-fuelled, or a third in a position you can't keep. Fix those and the story changes.

Equipment helps most when it's simple. Tyres and pressure are free speed if you stop guessing. Modern tubeless clinchers at sensible pressures beat narrow, rock-hard setups on real roads. Too hard and you skip across bumps; too soft and you squirm. Start with the brand's chart and tune by feel for grip and comfort. An aero helmet helps if it fits and you can keep your head still. A fancy visor means nothing if your neck gives up after an hour. Clothing matters more than most admit — a tidy jersey is faster than a flappy one. On the bike itself, your fit is worth more than a new crank. Saddle height and fore–aft that let you extend without rocking; reach you can hold without shrugging; bar width that matches your shoulders so you can breathe. A "fit" you can hold for twenty minutes is not a fit. It's a pose. Coach's note: Buy simplicity that makes your day easier. Ignore complexity that makes you feel fast on Instagram.

Course and conditions beat ego. Learn your race profile. Where are the long false flats where pacing goes to die? Where must you eat by time, not feel? If wind builds late, temper ambition early. If heat is a factor, accept slower numbers and focus on cooling and intake. A "perfect plan" that ignores weather is a story, not a strategy. Recon if you can. If you can't, simulate the shape locally: mimic climb distribution and practise fuelling at the same time points. Write three lines you'll use on the day and commit them to memory: Fuel early. Cadence is control. Finish clean. Not poetry. Instructions.

Bricks, progressed gently, change everything. Start short. Normalise the feeling. Build control only once calm is automatic. Weeks 1–2: 45–60 minutes Zone 2 ride → 8–10 minutes very easy run. Goal: make the shift ordinary. Weeks 3–4: 60–75 minutes ride with 2 × 10 minutes steady → 12–15 minutes easy, last 3–5 steady. Goal: learn restraint. Weeks 5–6: 75–90 minutes ride with 3 × 10 steady → 15–20 minutes run starting easy, building to intended race feel for 5 minutes. Goal: practise the settle. Weeks 7–8: 90 minutes ride with 20–30 minute blocks at race-like effort and fuelling on schedule → 20 minutes run (first 5 easy, next 10 controlled pace, last 5 easy). Goal: hold form with real inputs. If life is loud, keep the run short and honest. Consistency beats bravado.

Indoors, control the controllables: big fan, bottles in reach, towel ready. Calibrate your trainer the same way each time; consistency beats absolute accuracy. Use erg mode for steady work if it helps; use resistance mode for threshold and above so cadence and rhythm are yours. Outdoors, pick roads that match the work. Out-and-back beats stop-start loops when you need even pacing. If lights and traffic break the rhythm, accept it and ride easier rather than forcing numbers that don't belong there.

Mental skills make watts useful. Your head unit can show lap power; it can't tell you what to do with your next breath. Keep cues short and repeatable. On strength segments: tall torso, quiet hips, smooth pressure. On sweet spot: breathe low, elbows soft, even power. On the long ride: fuel early, sit still, finish clean. On the brick: calm cadence into calm feet. Decide one adjustment you'll make if today isn't your day. "If power won't hold cleanly, I cut the interval by two minutes and keep form." "If heat spikes, I reduce by five watts and drink now." Decide before you start; save the drama for someone else's file. Coach's note: Fewer stories. More decisions.

Strength away from the bike holds your posture together and makes hour three feel like hour one. Keep it simple: hinge (Romanian deadlift or good morning) for posterior chain in aero; split squat or step-up for single-leg control; row or pulldown for upper-back posture and relaxed shoulders; carry (suitcase or farmer) for anti-sway hips. Two sets of 6–10 controlled reps. Twice a week in base, once in season. Full range. One rep left in the tank. You're training positions and force paths, not chasing a deadlift PB. Pair it with five minutes of activation before key rides: hip openers, band pull-aparts, a few gentle standing accelerations to wake the pattern.

When you're blank, use clean templates and get on with it. Sweet-Spot Builder: 10–15 easy → 3 × 12 at high Z3/low Z4 (5 easy) → 10 down.

Strength-Endurance Ladder: 10 easy → 4/6/8/6/4 min at Z3, 55–60 rpm (3 easy) → 10 down.

High-Cadence Sharpen: 10 easy → 3 × (6 min Z2 + 6 × 20 s spin-up / 40 s easy) → 10 down.

Race-Prep Progression: 30 Z2 → 2 × 20 min high Z2/low Z3 (5 easy) → 20 Z2 → 10–15 easy run.

Brick Calmer: 60 Z2 with 3 × 5 min steady → transition → 12 min run (6 very easy, 6 steady).

Progress by adding a rep, nudging time, or trimming rest. If form goes, volume waits.

If you keep only a few lines from this chapter, keep these. Cycling isn't about peak power; it's about sustainable output. Train how you'll race; don't race your training. Efficiency, posture, and pacing — that's free speed.

Pause & apply: Pick one ride this week and give it a single purpose and two cues. Stage your bottle and fuel before you clip in. Add a brick run you can finish clean. Shift early on the first hill. Keep your head still on the first tailwind. Eat before you feel clever. Ride like you intend to run.

You don't need to be the strongest cyclist in your age group. You need to be the smartest one on race day.

Chapter 7 – Running: Speed, Threshold & Endurance

If your plan makes you dread lacing up, it's not you — it's the plan. Running shouldn't feel like guessing, or like every session is a punishment dressed as "grit." Done well, it's structured and direct. It has rhythm. Some days it's even enjoyable. The goal here isn't to turn you into a metronome. It's to give you a way of running that suits your life, builds fitness you can actually use, and keeps you healthy enough to keep going. The frame is simple: speed for sharpness, threshold for control, endurance for durability. You don't need all three every day. You do need a steady rotation that respects recovery and respects your calendar. Build those pieces in the right order, and running starts to feel like something you know how to do — not something you survive.

Most runners go wrong in the same places. They turn "easy" into "medium because it feels respectable." They turn "threshold" into an audition for race day. They treat long runs like badges rather than training. They try to live on motivation rather than systems. Then they wonder why little pains keep getting louder and pace stops moving. The fix is not heroic. It's clarity and sequence: sharpen, control, endure — with space between the hard days so your body can do what it's very good at when you let it: adapt.

Speed first, because it sets your movement pattern. Speed doesn't mean wild sprints and photos of agony. It means short, crisp work that cleans up mechanics and wakes the nervous system. Think 6–10 × 10–20 seconds of strides with full recovery, hill sprints that teach you to push the ground away with a tall posture, and drills that make your feet and hips talk to each other. You're not chasing splits on these; you're chasing feel: quick but relaxed, tall but soft, snappy but quiet. Put speed on a day when you're fresh and you'll feel it feed the rest of the week.

Threshold next, because it's the bridge between fast and far. Threshold is controlled hard — a place you can hold for a long interval with steady breathing and steady form, not a place you cling to with your teeth. If you can chat freely, you're too easy. If you can't finish a complete sentence between breaths, you're too hard. The sweet spot sits in that "I could keep this up, but I will definitely notice it" band. Get this right and race pace stops feeling like a cliff edge and starts feeling like a gear. Most runners overcook it. The cure is boring: even splits, small recoveries, repeatable sets. Let the watch report; let your breath decide.

Endurance sits under everything. Long runs are not punishment. They are where you rehearse patience, fuelling, and form under gentle fatigue. Some will be purely easy, some will finish stronger, and some will carry short race-pace segments. The type you choose depends on where you are in the season and what you're training for. None of them should flatten you for three days. If they do, your long run has become the race of your week. Scale it, tidy it, or change its purpose.

Mark learned this the hard way. He wanted a 1:30 half marathon. He doubled down on miles and "threshold," which was actually race pace with hope. He ran every day because he felt he should. He plateaued, then sagged. We cut his weekly volume by a fifth, gave him a real easy day, separated speed from threshold, and wrote threshold like a professional would: controlled, even. He ran 1:29:22. More importantly, he said he liked running again. The time was nice. The sustainability was the actual win.

Let's make this practical and keep the tone you've seen in the swim and bike chapters: flowing, clear, repeatable. Running is coordination under load. Start each quality session with five to eight minutes of movement that wakes what you need: ankle rocks, hip openers, skips (A and B if you know them), a few short drills or strides. End each with two quiet minutes — easy jog or walk — so you leave the session with form, not chaos. If the first kilometre of any run sets the whole tone, set that kilometre on purpose: slower than you think, posture tall, arms low and quiet, breath low in the ribs. Most "bad" runs are rescued by a calmer first five minutes.

Shoes and terrain shape how your legs feel tomorrow. Reserve your light, snappy shoes for faster or shorter sessions. Use stable, forgiving trainers for volume. If you move every run to cambered roads or lumpy trails, your hips will tell you about it. Vary surfaces. Asphalt for rhythm. Trail for strength and patience. Track sparingly unless you're already resilient; it's honest and it's harsh. If a treadmill saves your week, use it — set 1–2% gradient for feel, don't yank the side rails, keep your posture tall.

Cadence is often a by-product of good form, not a number to force. If you try to hit 180 at any cost, you'll scramble. Instead, shorten the step a touch when tired, keep feet landing under you rather than ahead, and aim for quiet contacts. Don't chase a number; chase silence and symmetry.

Breath cues keep you honest when the watch argues. On easy runs: in for three, out for three, or in for three, out for two if you prefer. On threshold: breathing is firmer but rhythmic; if you're gasping, you're racing. On speed: breathe low, not high; you're moving fast, not panicking. If you can't find your breath, slow to a walk for thirty seconds, collect it, and restart. You didn't lose — you reset.

Fuel quietly decides how your running goes. Anything over 75–90 minutes wants a plan. Eat something simple 60–90 minutes before. Carry fluid if heat or duration demands it. On long runs with work inside, aim small sips often. Practice gels if you'll race with them. Learn which ones agree with you. Write it down. Most blow-ups start as decisions you didn't make before you left the door.

Strength and mobility don't need a new life. Twice a week in base, once in season: hinges (RDLs), split squats, calf raises, single-leg balance with reach, a pull (row), a push (push-up), and carries. Full range, no grinding, stop with one rep in the tank. Add simple footwork: towel scrunches, short barefoot drills on grass if your feet tolerate it, and daily ankle circles. Your calves are your springs; treat them that way.

Simple, Repeatable Running Week (Mon–Sun)

Monday — Rest / Mobility / Light Strength (10–30 min) Keep it easy: ankle rocks, hip openers, T-spine rotations, 1–2 sets of split squats, RDLs, calf raises, and a row or push-up. Aim: keep tissues happy; make positions available. Win line: nothing is sore tomorrow.

Tuesday — Threshold With Control (50–70 min) Warm 10–15 min easy → 4–6 × 15–20 s strides, walk/easy jog back. Main set (pick one):

3 × 10 min @ threshold, 2–3 min easy jog, or

4 × 8 min @ threshold, 2 min easy. Cool 10 min easy. Aim: even effort, calm breathing, posture that lasts. Cues: tall ribcage, elbows low, relax jaw. Win line: last rep matches the first within a few seconds.

Wednesday — Easy Aerobic + Optional Form Touch (35–60 min) All Z2 conversational. Optional: finish with 4 × 15 s relaxed strides (only if you feel fresh). Aim: aerobic support + recovery from Tuesday. Win line: you'd happily keep going 10 more minutes.

Thursday — Speed + Aerobic (45–60 min) Warm 15 min easy + mobility. Drills 2–4 min (skips, high knees, butt kicks, straight-leg bounds). Main set: 8–10 × 15–20 s strides @ 5K effort or faster, 60–90 s easy jog between. Flow straight into 15–25 min easy-aerobic. Aim: sharpen mechanics, then bank relaxed volume. Cues: quick but quiet; land under you; arms short and smooth. Win line: strides feel snappy without strain; easy block truly easy.

Friday — Rest / Mobility / Light Strength (10–30 min) Same menu as Monday (or swap in single-leg balance, carries, gentle core). Aim: maintain the chassis; arrive fresh for Saturday. Win line: you feel primed, not tired.

Saturday — Long Run (70–120+ min, context-dependent) Rotate across weeks:

Easy long: all Z2, conversational.

Progression: final third a touch firmer, still within conversation breath.

Race-pace bites: 3 × 8–10 min at goal pace w/ 5 min easy, or a 20–30 min controlled-hard block (HM/M prep). Start slower than you think for 10–15 min. Fuel, especially if you include work. Aim: durability, patience, fuelling practice. Cues: soft feet, long back, quiet shoulders. Win line: you finish knowing you could have done more.

Sunday — Optional Easy Shuffle (20–40 min) or Rest If the week was heavy, take the win and rest.

When life compresses your week

Two runs? Defend Tuesday (threshold) and Saturday (long).
Three runs? Add Thursday (speed + aerobic).
If you're squeezed, move Thursday's strides into Tuesday's warm-up (4–6 instead of 8–10) and sprinkle 10–15 min easy onto one other day.

If you must shift the long run, keep ≥1 easy day between threshold and long.

Progress (every 4–6 weeks, only if last reps look like first)

Add one threshold rep or extend each by ~1 min — not both.

Long run: extend by 10–15 min every other week (if sleep/fuel are solid).

Every 3rd–4th week, drop volume 15–25% and keep one short quality touch (e.g., 2 × 8 min threshold) so freshness can catch you.

Small but key notes

Warm-up rule: the first kilometre is deliberately slow. Set posture and breath.

Fuel: >75–90 min wants a plan. Eat 60–90 min before; sip during longer/hot runs; practise race carbs if you'll use them.

Shoes: rotate a daily trainer + a lighter pair for quality to spread load.

Terrain: vary surfaces; use short hill sprints (6–8 × 8–12 s, full walk back) occasionally on speed weeks.

Debrief: 2 lines after key sessions → Feel + Lesson. Patterns > vibes.

Coach's note: Scale before you scrap. The version that protects the week beats the perfect plan you abandon. Finish clean.

Three versions of the same week so it survives real life: Plan A (as drawn): Tue threshold, Thu speed + aerobic, Sat long, Sun easy/rest. Plan B (work exploded): Keep Tue as 3 × 8 minutes instead of 3 × 10; Thu becomes 6 strides inside a 35-minute easy run; Sat long trimmed by 15–20 minutes with fuelling still practiced; Sun rest. Plan C (sleep collapsed): Tue becomes 30–40 easy with 4 strides; Thu is 2 × 6 minutes controlled with 2 minutes easy if you feel good, else easy; Sat 60–75 easy with 2 × 6 minutes at "steady, not hard;" Sun off. Habit intact, load reduced.

Terrain and hills are tools, not traps. Use short hill sprints (6–8 × 8–12 seconds, full walk back) on some speed days to build power with low injury risk. Use moderate hills in long runs to teach patience and posture. Keep steep descents short unless your quads already like them; soreness is not training. If you're training for a hilly race, copy the shape: include long gentle climbs in long runs and put small controlled efforts at the top to learn not to collapse after the crest.

Pacing and watches need boundaries. For threshold, choose looped or out-and-back routes you know. If heat or wind skew the numbers, let RPE lead and use heart rate as "is this appropriately hard" rather than "hit 4:18/km no matter what." If you find yourself arguing with your watch every kilometre, switch to lap pace or hide pace entirely and let your breath steer. You can always look at the file after. The point in the moment is control, not a screenshot.

Cues keep you from overthinking. Keep two per run. Examples: tall/soft for easy. Even/quiet for threshold. Short/quick for strides. If your mind wanders, that's fine. If it wanders to catastrophes, come back to your feet — are they quiet? Are they landing under you? These small anchors beat long speeches.

Common problems, useful fixes: Easy isn't easy. Make it social, leave the watch, or cap heart rate to a number you can actually keep. If you can't speak in phrases, you're too fast. Threshold turns into a race. Pre-write the set and the first kilometre pace you'll not exceed. If you miss a rep, cut the next by a minute and keep quality. Calves keep tightening. Add calf raises (straight and bent knee), reduce abrupt changes in shoe stack height, and keep strides short the first week you switch surfaces. Shins talk on downhills. Shorten step, land under you, choose softer surfaces for a fortnight, and add anterior tibialis work (toe raises). Hips ache after long runs. Add split squats and lateral work (band walks). Ease cambered roads. Check that you're not leaning from the waist. Always fading late. Eat earlier. Start slower. Add short "steady" segments earlier in the long run rather than only at the end. • Niggle brewing. Trade the next hard run for 30–40 minutes easy or bike, keep strength, and re-test after 48 hours. Ending clean beats pushing for one more rep.

Shoes: rotate at least two pairs if you can — one daily trainer, one lighter pair for quality. It spreads load and changes the stress pattern week to week. Replace when the midsole feels dead rather than when the outsole looks worn; your legs feel foam before your eyes spot wear.

Heat and cold change the rules. In heat, slow by feel, reduce threshold length a touch, and drink. In cold, extend your warm-up and don't chase pace on frozen paths. If a storm or a heat wave rolls through, this is not you going soft; it's you training intelligently.

Racing is just training with timing. Build race-pace familiarity inside threshold weeks: marathoners might run 20–30 minutes at goal pace inside a long run every other week for a block; half-marathoners can use 3 × 10–12 minutes at goal pace with short jogs; 10K runners can sprinkle 5 × 5 minutes at 10K feel with 2 minutes easy. Keep the work tidy. If your last repeat is an audition, you're too hot. Save that appetite for the day.

Run bricks matter for triathletes, and we've already talked about them on the bike side. Here's the handshake from the run side: your first kilometre off the bike is about calming your stride. Let your cadence find you; don't fight for length. Think quiet feet, long exhale. If you insist on "goal pace" in the first two minutes, you'll go there — and you'll spend the next twenty paying for it. Build in, then hold. That's how negative splits happen in real life.

Data can help if it stays in its lane. One intent per session. One or two metrics only. RPE and breath for live steering. Pace and splits for debrief. If you love charts, look at trends every two to four weeks, not daily. If you hate charts, keep a ledger: five lines once a week — sessions started on time, nights of 7+ hours, instances of honest easy, times you fuelled before you faded, one decision you're proud of that won't show on Strava. Quiet evidence beats noisy apps.

Strength of mind isn't a motivational speech. It's a habit. Decide your adjustment before you start: "If the second threshold rep feels off, I cut the third by two minutes and keep shape." "If my knee speaks on hills, I move to flatter ground today." When the decision is made in advance, there's no drama to chew on mid-run. You just do the version that keeps the season moving.

A simple 6–8 week progression you can drop into most base-to-build blocks: Weeks 1–2: Threshold 3 × 8 minutes (2 easy), strides 8–10 × 15 s, long run easy. Weeks 3–4: Threshold 3 × 10 minutes (2–3 easy), strides as before, long run progression last 20–30 minutes steady. Weeks 5–6: Threshold 4 × 8 minutes (2 easy) or 2 × 15 minutes (3 easy), strides with 2–3 short hill sprints, long run with 20–30 min at race feel. Weeks 7–8: Lighter volume: threshold touch as 2 × 8 minutes, strides cut to 6–8, long run shorter and easy. Reassess notes and adjust zones by feel, not by one hero day.

And because you'll ask: yes, treadmill is fine. Keep the first two minutes a walk-to-jog ramp, use a small incline for feel, don't stare at your knees. If you're doing threshold on a treadmill, use time and breath, not pace alone; machines lie differently on different days. If you can, ventilate the room. Heat creep will change your heart rate and story.

Finally, recover on purpose. Eat something within an hour — protein and carbs — then normal meals. Swap ten mindless minutes on your phone for ten mindful minutes with a foam roller or, better, on the floor doing nothing while your heart rate comes down. When life is noisy, that is your reset. If you slept poorly, your priority is not making up a session; it's protecting the next two. Running rewards humility faster than bravado.

If you keep only a handful of lines from this chapter, keep these. Easy means easy; that's where you build the base. Threshold is controlled hard; it teaches you to race. Speed is short and crisp; it keeps you moving well. Use each on purpose. Don't race your training. Stack small wins; they compound. Write two lines after each run: feel and lesson. Then get on with your day.

Pause & apply: choose two cues for your next run. Decide your adjustment rule before you leave. Put one gel in your pocket for the next long run and set a reminder to use it. Add 4–6 strides at the end of an easy run this week and notice how the first kilometre of the next day feels. Small hinges; big doors.

You don't need to run more to become a runner who races well. You need to run with intention, hold your shape when it matters, and keep enough in the tank to come back tomorrow. That's how we build seasons that last and results that show up on time.

Chapter 8 – Strength: Stability, Movement & Athlete Muscle

Strength training doesn't make you bulky or slow. Skipping it makes you fragile. If you're piling hours into swim, bike, and run but your hips wobble, your ankles jam, and your shoulders complain, you're building fitness on a shaky frame. This chapter is the fix — no bodybuilding templates, no "three sets of everything forever," no noise. Just what transfers: stable joints, clean movement, useful muscle. Strong isn't a look. It's a foundation.

The point is simple: your engine only helps if the chassis can carry it. Strength work is how you keep positions, create force without leaking it, and hold form when the session or the race gets loud. It isn't optional conditioning you "add if there's time." It's the thing that makes all the rest more repeatable.

Most endurance athletes make the same mistake. They avoid strength until they're forced into it by a niggle, then panic-lift random circuits until the pain quiets down, then stop again. Or they chase "functional" fluff that looks athletic and does nothing. The fix isn't complicated. It's a short list done well, week after week: move well, load well, spring a little, and brace the middle. Let's build that, clean and calm, and make it fit your life.

Start with movement, not load. If your ankles won't bend, your knees and hips will do their job and everyone else's. If your hips can't extend, your lower back will volunteer. If your shoulder blades don't glide, your neck and rotator cuff will pay. You don't need to become a mobility hobbyist. You need the ranges that your sports demand, available on demand.

Ankles: you want knee-over-toe range without the heel popping. Ten slow knee drives over the big toe and little toe each side before key runs and rides is enough. Hips: you want extension without lumbar sway and rotation without collapsing the knee. Couch stretch, 90/90 rotations, and a few tall-kneel hip extensions get you there. Shoulders: you want the blade to slide and tip so the arm can reach without the neck doing the work. Band Y-T-W, wall slides, and a few light pulldowns set the path.

None of this is a warm-up performance. Two to five minutes before the session you actually care about, then go and lift or go and run. Movement gives you access. Strength locks it in.

Coach's note: Mobility is permission. Strength is ownership.

Now the meat: strength. You don't need an encyclopaedia of lifts. You need a hinge, a squat pattern, a push, a pull, and a carry. That's it. Choose the versions you can learn quickly, load safely, and recover from while you still swim, bike, and run.

Hinge: Romanian deadlift (dumbbells or bar) or trap-bar deadlift. Teaches you to load the posterior chain without folding in half. Squat pattern: split squat or rear-foot-elevated (Bulgarian) split squat. Single-leg on purpose — it looks more like your sports and keeps egos tidy. Push: push-up progression or incline dumbbell press. You don't need a barbell bench to hold aero or stroke water. Pull: one-arm row and pulldown/chin-up (assisted if needed). This is posture and shoulder health under fatigue. Carry: suitcase carry or farmer carry. Breathing and bracing while you move — anti-sway hips in disguise.

Do these in full ranges with control. Lower with intention, pause when needed to find the position, and drive like you mean it — without a face you'd regret on camera. Three to four lifts per session, two to four sets each, six to ten reps when building, three to six reps when peaking strength in the off-season. Leave one rep in the tank. Finish with 5–8 minutes of core that resists motion, not endless sit-ups:

dead bugs, side planks, palloff presses, tall-kneel chops and lifts.

Coach's note: "Full range at a weight you can own" beats "heavier, messier" every day of a long season.

Elasticity matters, because running and fast cycling aren't slow grinds; they're bounce and rhythm. You don't need to turn yourself into a jumper. You do need to remind your tissues they're springs. Think of two short doses a week in build phases, once a week in-season, and none if tissues complain. Keep contacts low, volumes small, and recoveries honest.

Low-dose plyos: pogos (two-foot ankle hops), line hops (forward/back, side/side), low box step-offs to small jumps, and very short shallow bounds. Ten to twenty ground contacts per drill, two to three drills total. Stop while it still looks good. Med-ball: chest pass to wall, overhead throw, rotational throw. Three to five sets of three to five crisp reps. Rest between like you mean it. Resisted sprint primers: light band or slight uphill, 4–6 × 8–12 seconds. This is technique and intent, not max output.

If your calves or Achilles tend to talk, build basic calf strength first: straight-knee and bent-knee raises, two to three sets of 8–15 each, three to five second lowers, full range. Then add mild plyos weeks later.

Core is not crunches. Your sports ask you to keep a long spine while your limbs pull and push, breathe while you brace, and resist rotation and extension rather than perform them. Train that.

Anti-extension: dead bugs, hollow variations, rollouts if tolerated. Anti-rotation: palloff press holds and step-outs, half-kneel cable chops. Anti-lateral-flexion: suitcase carries, side planks with top-leg march. Integration: tall-kneel overhead presses, split-stance rows and pushes.

Two or three drills, 30–45 seconds or 6–10 controlled reps, two sets is plenty if the lifts already taxed you. The measure isn't tremble; it's control.

Coach's note: If you can't breathe, you're not bracing — you're holding your breath.

What this actually looks like in a week depends on your phase and your life. Keep it boring on paper and sharp in practice.

Off-season (2–3 sessions/week, 35–55 minutes each)

Session A: hinge (RDL), split squat, one-arm row, push-up/push, suitcase carry, anti-rotation.

Session B: trap-bar deadlift or heavier hinge, rear-foot-elevated split squat (lighter, more range), pulldown/chin variation, incline press, farmer carry, anti-extension.

Optional C (short): med-ball throws + low-dose plyos + carries + quick mobility.

Progress by adding a set, nudging load 2–5 kg or trimming tempo slightly — one change at a time. If swim/bike/run volume is also rising, progress slower.

In-season (1–2 sessions/week, 20–35 minutes)

Session A (maintenance): hinge, split squat, one pull, one push, one carry, one core. Two sets each, 6–8 reps, leave a rep in the tank.

Session B (optional, micro): 12–18 minutes of med-ball + carries + core after an easy session or before a rest day.

Brick-integrated options (8–15 minutes)

Before run: activation (glute bridge, band lateral steps, calf raises, palloff press), then go.

After bike: 2 rounds of 3 moves (RDL light, split squat, row) 2 × 6–8 each, slow lowers, then short easy run.

This is not decorative. It's putting strength where it tilts the week in your favour.

Rachel's rebuild is the template for when things have come apart. She spent a season bouncing between hamstring tightness and calf strains. Raced once. Sat twice. Felt cursed. We stopped running for four weeks. Bikes and swims stayed, gently. Strength became the spine: isometric hamstring bridges and split-stance holds, single-leg RDLs to mid-shin, step-downs for eccentric patellar load, hip airplanes against the wall for control, tib raises for the shins, short foot work. We progressed slow, not because caution is a personality trait, but because tissues adapt to the forces you ask of them consistently, not dramatically.

Week five she jogged every other day: ten minutes easy, then walk, then ten more, then stop. Week six we added strides and a little hill. Week eight she ran four days a week, kept one strength session, and we didn't let her win arguments with pace for a month. Three months in she was back to full volume and setting bests, not because she found the perfect shoe, but because her joints had a plan and her tissues had time.

Coach's note: Return-to-run is a strength plan wearing trainers.

Let's write the same kind of strength week you saw in swim and bike — clear, repeatable, and adjustable.

Monday — Strength 1 (full-body, 35–45 min)

Prep (3–5 min): ankle rocks ×10/side, 90/90 hips ×6/side, band Y-T-W ×8 each.

Main:

Hinge: Romanian deadlift 3 × 6–8 (3 seconds down, 1 second up).

Split squat (rear foot elevated): 3 × 6–8/side (pause one second at the bottom).

Row (one-arm): 3 × 8–10/side.

Push-up or incline DB press: 3 × 6–10.

Suitcase carry: 2 × 20–30 m/side (upright, slow).

Core finisher: dead bug 2 × 8/side (slow), palloff press hold 2 × 20–30 s/side.

Thursday — Strength 2 (power/elasticity + strength, 25–35 min)

Prep (3 min): light pogo practice 2 × 10, calf raise 2 × 10 (3 seconds down).

Power: med-ball chest pass 4 × 3, rotational throw 4 × 3/side (rest 45–60 s).

Main (reduced volume):

Trap-bar deadlift or goblet squat 3 × 4–6 (crisp, own the rep).

Pulldown/chin (assisted okay) 3 × 5–8.

Lateral band walk 2 × 12–15/side.

Core/carry: side plank 2 × 20–30 s/side, farmer carry 2 × 20–30 m.

Saturday — Activation micro (8–12 min before long bike/run)

Glute bridge 2 × 10 (1 second hold).

Band lateral step 2 × 12/side.

Calf raise 2 × 12 (straight knee).

Palloff press 2 × 20 s/side.

Daily — Reset (5 minutes, optional)

Thoracic extension over foam roller ×6–8.

Hip flexor stretch 1 × 30–45 s/side.

Two long exhales lying on your back, feet up, to downshift.

If life explodes, keep a single 20–30-minute strength session and the 8–12 minute activation before one key endurance session. That alone changes how your week feels.

Progress over 4–6 weeks by adding one set on the main lifts or nudging load slightly. Then take a lighter week: halves sets or drop one main lift, keep activation and core. You don't detrain in five days. You consolidate.

Three versions of the same week so it survives real life: Plan A (as drawn): Mon + Thu + Sat micro. Plan B (work exploded): One 25–30 min session midweek with hinge, split squat, row, carry, and a core pair. Keep the Sat micro. Plan C (sleep collapsed): Two 12–18 min micro-sessions (Mon/Sat) of activation + one main lift + carries, everything else floats.

Coach's note: The best strength plan is the one you repeat. The glamorous one you skip doesn't count.

How heavy is heavy? Heavy enough that the last two reps make you pay attention to posture, but not so heavy the rep changes shape. If a set looks like a different exercise from the first rep to the last, the weight is lying to you. Move the barbell or dumbbell with intent. Lower with control, feel end range, stand or pull with speed you can keep. Tempo is a tool: slower lowers teach position, faster intent on the way up teaches you to produce force. Don't mix them randomly.

Where does strength go around key endurance sessions? If Tuesday is threshold run and Thursday is sweet-spot bike, put Strength 1 on Monday, Strength 2 on Thursday before an easier spin or after threshold if you know you tolerate it. Avoid heavy lower body the day before your long run until you know your recovery speed. In race week, keep a micro-dose 3–5 days out: 2 × 3–4 reps on hinge and split squat at ~70% of normal load, one pull, one carry, and go home.

What about sore? You're allowed to feel like you lifted. You're not allowed to sabotage the swim/bike/run you care about. If muscle soreness bleeds into form, you overdid it. Pull 20–30% next time, or move the session to a different day.

Common problems, useful fixes:

Knees cave on squats/split squats: widen stance slightly, think "press the floor apart," reduce load, use a small band above knees as a reminder, not a crutch.

Hinge becomes a back bend: soften knees, push hips back to the wall, keep ribs down, slide the weight down the front of the thighs. If you can't feel hamstrings, it's too low or too loose.

Shoulders shrug in rows and pushes: exhale, pack the shoulder blades gently down and back, think long neck, lighten the weight.

Carries tilt into a list: go lighter and slower, set the pelvis under you, ribs stacked over pelvis, walk as if you're balancing a glass on your head.

Core = face strain: if you can't breathe during a plank, you're holding your breath. Drop the time, get your breath back, rebuild.

Plyos sting: stop. You're not late to elasticity. Build calf capacity, try low pogo contacts only, or remove plyos for a block.

Shoes and surfaces count in the gym, too. Lifting in squishy cushioned trainers makes balance work harder than it needs to be. Go barefoot or wear something flat and firm if it's safe and allowed. For split squats, a slider or towel under the back foot can reduce fuss. For carries, space matters more than weight; find a line you can walk without weaving through a crowd.

Equipment is secondary. Dumbbells, a trap bar, a cable stack, a few bands, a med-ball. If you don't have a trap bar, heavy Kettlebell RDLs or two dumbbells work. If you don't have a cable, use a band for palloff and chops. If you don't have a bench, use the floor and a pair of boxes. Buy simplicity that gets used. Ignore complexity that looks clever on social media.

Coach's note: Tools don't make the plan. The plan makes the tools useful.

Strength for swimmers, cyclists, and runners looks the same underneath but gets expressed slightly differently.

Swim lens: upper-back strength and shoulder control buy you water feel and reduce tug-of-war with the neck. Rows and pulldowns matter; so do serratus-friendly pushes (incline, push-up plus). Don't chase massive paddles in the weight room; chase blades that move. Finish with thoracic mobility so you can breathe without shrugging.

Bike lens: hinges and carries keep you honest in aero. Single-leg work and isometrics (long split-squat holds) teach you to produce force without rolling the pelvis. Light hip flexor work (banded marches) helps position, not power. Core anti-rotation keeps you steady in crosswinds.

Run lens: calves and feet get their own paragraph. Heavy-ish straight-knee calf raises and bent-knee soleus raises, two to three sets of 6–10 slow reps each, change how your lower legs feel at 90 minutes. Add isometric holds (30–45 seconds mid-range) once a week. Pair with low-dose plyos only when the basics are easy. Hips: split squats and lateral work (band walks) pay off on hills and in the last third of races. Don't skip them because they're not Instagram.

How to progress without drama:

Range → tempo → load → complexity. Earn the next step.

Add a set before you add load if technique still wobbles.

Trim rest only when you don't need it, not to make the session feel "harder."

Every fourth week, pull volume or load ~20% and keep quality.

After illness, return at 60–70% of last comfortable load and rebuild in two weeks, not two days.

If you're in a heavy endurance week or you went long by accident, adjust strength: drop one main lift and carry on. If you've slept badly two nights in a row, skip heavy hinge and do light range work and carries. The point isn't to prove you can do everything at once. It's to keep the season moving.

Nutrition around strength is straightforward. Eat something with protein and carbs within an hour. If you lift before a key session, keep the lift short and arrive fed. If you lift after, eat before you get distracted. Hydrate. If you cramp in the gym, you didn't discover a new weakness — you discovered you were under-fuelled.

Recovery is not a spa day. It's you deciding to stop before your form dies, you sleeping on purpose, and you keeping five minutes of mobility in the bank daily so positions don't disappear between sessions. Foam roll if it helps your head. It won't lengthen your hamstrings. Your choices will.

Templates you can use when you're blank:

30-minute maintenance (hotel gym version)

RDL 3 × 6–8

Rear-foot-elevated split squat 2 × 6–8/side

One-arm row 2 × 8–10/side

Push-up 2 × 6–10

Suitcase carry 2 × 20–30 m/side (If time: palloff press 2 × 20 s/side)

Power touch (15–20 minutes)

Med-ball chest pass 4 × 3 (rest 45–60 s)

Rotational throw 4 × 3/side

Pogo 2 × 10

Farmer carry 2 × 30 m

Foot & calf pack (12–15 minutes, runners)

Straight-knee calf raise 3 × 8 (3 seconds down)

Bent-knee calf raise 3 × 8

Tib raise 2 × 12–15

Short-foot holds 3 × 20 s

Core anti-everything (10–12 minutes)

Dead bug 2 × 8/side

Side plank 2 × 20–30 s/side

Palloff press step-out 2 × 6/side

Tall-kneel overhead press 2 × 6

Use one. Move on.

If you only keep a few lines from this chapter, keep these. Strength isn't extra; it's essential. You don't need to train like a lifter; you need to train like an athlete. Full range, controlled tempo, one rep in the tank. Hinge, split squat, row, press, carry, brace — every week, in small, repeatable doses. Elasticity is a seasoning, not a meal. Strong joints are fast joints. Strong positions make hard days feel normal.

Pause & apply: schedule two strength touches next week — one 35–45 minute full-body and one 10–15 minute activation. Choose your hinge and your split-squat load you can own. Add calf work if you run, one carry if you bike, one pulldown if you swim. Write one rule on your plan: stop when the shape breaks. Then keep showing up. Small, tidy bricks build big, durable walls.

Chapter 9 – Your Season: Building, Peaking & Performing

Training without a season is like building without a blueprint. You can stack bricks for months and call it "work", but the wall won't be straight and it won't be there when you need it. A good year has rhythm. It has phases that lift you up, phases that calm you down, and edges that sharpen at the right time. It also has breathing room, because life doesn't read your plan.

This chapter gives you the shape. Not commandments— just a frame you can live inside. You'll see how to move from general to specific, how to put races in places that make sense, how to taper without unravelling, and how to keep confidence while you adjust for travel, illness, and the unexpected. The aim is simple: a year that makes sense while you're in it and delivers when it counts.

Most athletes plan in bursts. They circle two or three races, throw themselves at training like a January clean-eating kick, then try to hold that gear for months. It's reactive. It burns bright, then dims. Smart seasons are proactive. They respect how bodies adapt: stress, absorb, sharpen, express. If you've ever felt permanently "almost ready", you've met a year without phases. Let's fix that.

At Smart Performance we talk about five jobs your year must do, and we give each job a phase. The labels are less important than the decisions they change. First you reset, because endings deserve an exhale. Then you build a base, because foundations come before storeys. Then you build on purpose, because specificity is where fitness becomes performance. Then you peak, because sharpening is not the same as searching. Then you perform and recover, because a race is not the end; it's a hinge to the next beginning.

Reset is short and human. You step away from shoulds. You sleep like you mean it. You check the niggles you've been ignoring. You move, but lightly. You write a few lines about what worked, what didn't, and what to change. It might be two weeks after a half marathon. It might be a long weekend after a heavy build. The point isn't the calendar; it's the exhale. Coach's note: recovery isn't what you earn after perfection—it's the permission that lets you keep going.

Base is steady and patient. Aerobic volume grows. Strength is consistent. Skills sit front and centre: timing in the water, posture on the bike, mechanics in the run. Intensity exists, but it's small and smart: strides, short hill sprints, a controlled dose of tempo that feels like control, not drama. You arrive at the end of a base block feeling hungry, not cooked. You miss sessions without a Greek chorus in your head. You return from a weekend away without believing you've "lost it". You're laying floorboards, not painting skirting boards.

Build is where the work gains teeth. Threshold becomes a weekly staple. Long rides or runs include segments where you practise pace under mild fatigue. Bricks grow from "so my legs remember" to "so my legs behave". Open water swims carry sighting and "fast-to-calm" starts. You don't throw your strength work away; you right-size it. You put a small race in the middle to learn, not to prove. The weeks have shape: stress that means something, recovery that actually recovers, notes that pay attention to feel as much as to data.

Peak is shorter than you think and calmer than you want. Volume comes down. Frequency stays. Intensity remains, but in small, tidy doses that feel like rehearsal rather than auditions. You practise race pace and then stop early while the shape is still good. You get specific without getting clever. You resist the urge to "top up" a decade's worth of fitness in ten days. You sleep. You list the three cues you'll use on the day and you rehearse them out loud.

Perform & recover is obvious and somehow still misunderstood. You execute. You eat like a human. You sleep. You write two short paragraphs about what went well and three practical changes you'll carry forward. You walk. You resist filling the quiet with new goals until you've listened to what the year just told you.

That loop—Reset, Base, Build, Peak, Perform—isn't a ladder. You'll circle through it more than once across twelve months. Sometimes with long versions. Sometimes with minis you fit around life. The trick is to let each phase do its job and to recognise the feeling when it's time to move on.

Dan is the neatest example of how a season turns a talented trier into a consistent racer. He trained in bursts, raced himself empty, then drifted until guilt pulled him back. He had two speeds: all-in and hiding. We mapped a year that matched his life rather than our fantasies. Winter: base with three strength touches a fortnight and swims that rebuilt his feel for water. Spring: a build that included one small local race to practise pacing and transitions without the pressure of perfection. Early summer: a short reset and a four-week speed block because his work went mad and his head needed variety. Autumn: a deliberate peak into his Ironman. It worked because it was paced like a story: set-up, development, climax, exhale. He hit both races, yes—but the real win was that he liked the months between.

You don't need Dan's exact calendar to get his outcome. You need his rhythm.

Start your season by pencilling anchors, not fantasies. Put your A-race down first. Put two possible B-races in the months before—events you can treat as dress rehearsals or stepping stones. Put your reset windows where real life demands them: the family holiday, the crunch month at work, the time of year you always pick up a cold. Work backwards from the A-race. Count weeks. Give each phase its space. And if the calendar refuses to cooperate, don't lie to yourself by squeezing a twelve-week build into four. Move the goal or change its size. There's more courage in a realistic plan than in heroic self-deception.

Now sketch the texture. A base month feels like this: you're training frequently, you're never crushed, and you're accumulating capacity. The long sessions are more about time than about speed. The "quality" is brief and tidy. You finish the month feeling like you could handle more. A build month feels like this: one or two sessions each week bite in a controlled way; the long sessions carry content rather than just volume; you practise pacing decisions; you learn from one event rather than judge yourself by it. A peak fortnight feels like this: sessions are shorter and sharper; your legs become springy again; you fiddle with your bike less; you worry that you're under-doing it; you go to bed anyway.

If you like numbers, give each phase its simple metrics. In base you might nudge run frequency from four days to five, hold weekly cycling between two and three rides, and keep swims smooth and skilful. In build you'll likely hold frequency while letting weekly load rise modestly, and you'll make your hard days actually hard and your easy days actually easy. In peak the numbers step back on paper while the quality remains. None of this needs to be neat. It does need to be intentional. Coach's note: if every month looks the same, you don't have a season—you have a loop.

There's a reason we like three weeks of work followed by one week lighter, or two-on, one-down when life is lively. Planned recovery beats accidental collapse. The lighter week still has a small taste of intensity, because speed disappears faster than endurance, but the total drops enough for freshness to catch you. Put those down weeks in your calendar now and protect them. If you only ever rest when you're wrecked, you'll always arrive late.

Taper deserves its own paragraph because this is where good plans panic. Sharpening is not stopping. It's keeping the frequency you're used to, reducing total volume by a sensible slice, and maintaining small doses of race-like work so your legs remember what they're for. Runners often settle well with ten to fourteen days: a first week where volume drops by a quarter and a second week where it falls again while strides and short race-pace segments keep rhythm alive. Triathletes tend to sit in a similar window: swims stay frequent with one controlled-hard taste, bikes include one early sweet-spot reminder and a midweek steady spin, runs include one short session where race cadence appears without strain. You will feel odd. You will doubt yourself. You will consider adding "just one more" hard thing. Don't. Taper feels like under-doing. That's the point. Let the work count.

You'll notice the same season can look different depending on the sport. A runner with a June half-marathon might float into January with easy volume and regular strength, build through spring with weekly threshold and long runs that alternate between purely easy and gently progressive, then sharpen for two to three weeks while sleep and confidence climb. They might use a March or April 10K as a B-race to practise pacing and learn how the new shoes feel at speed. After the half they'll step back for a week or two, then choose: do we play with short events through summer, or start laying the floorboards for an autumn marathon?

A triathlete with an August 70.3 might spend December and January rebuilding swim mechanics and holding strength at two or three touches a fortnight. February and March would layer in bike form work and gentle run threshold while long sessions widen. Spring becomes brick season—short and frequent at first, longer and more specific as the weeks pass. Early summer carries one or two race rehearsals: an Olympic-distance event you train through, or a local sprint where you practise transitions without the frenzy. July is the calm sharpening: shorter bricks, open-water confidence sets, nutrition rehearsed at race-like intakes. August executes. September breathes. October decides whether a short, playful block belongs before winter.

This is the same logic drawn in different colours: general to specific; teeth then polish; effort then ease.

When do you adjust? More often than you think, and sooner than you feel like you "should". The red flags are subtle and usually emotional before they become physical. If easy runs start to feel like chores, if heart rate is a notch high across a whole week at paces that were fine a fortnight ago, if you're short with people for no reason, if your long session has turned into a weekly epic followed by two days of swamp—those are early signs, not tests of grit. Pull one hard session. Add one early night. Eat more carbohydrates for forty-eight hours. Call a friend and go somewhere pretty at easy pace. The goal isn't to pass through pain; it's to stay in the game.

Niggles repeat their story with boring consistency: the same tendon speaks at the same mileage every Saturday; the same lower-back stiffness appears every time you do long turbo + brick; the same shoulder ache arrives every time you up paddle size. That's not fate. That's your plan showing you where it's out of tune. Adjust the stressor, not your expectations. Split the long session into two. Swap paddles for pull buoy while you rebuild catch feel. Trade a run for a bike for ten days. Most seasons are saved by small edits made early.

Travel, work spikes, and colds arrive on schedules of their own. A season survives because you expect them. Travel weeks can become "protect the anchors" weeks: one quality session done clean and one longer aerobic session that fits the logistics. Use the hotel gym to keep your positions (see the strength chapter's hotel template); fifteen minutes of carries and hinges stabilises more than you think. Work spikes deserve honesty: defend the session that most aligns with your phase and the long one that keeps your head and let the garnish go. Illness gets the simplest rule of all: above the neck and light = maybe; below the neck or fever = no. After fever, wait forty-eight hours and come back at sixty to seventy per cent for a few days. Fitness doesn't vanish. Impatience invites a sequel.

The fun part of planning is daydreaming about races; the useful part is deciding which ones matter. Not every event deserves the same treatment. Give your year one true A-race per season—or one across the whole year if it's a full marathon or an Ironman—and let everything else serve it. B-races become pencil sketches where you practise shoes, nutrition, or pacing without flaring your taper. C-races become hard sessions with number pins. When you label races this way, weeks become easier to write and easier to live. You stop tapering twelve times and wondering why you're always tired. You stop trying to prove yourself every month. You start learning on purpose.

If nerves rise during a peak—and they will—shrink the task. Bring it back to what you control this week: one quality session done cleanly; one long session finished with form; two nights of good sleep; one rehearsal of race cues; your kit list printed and annoyingly sensible. Confidence is not a feeling you wait for. It's the quiet result of clear actions repeated in view of your own eyes.

Coach's note: fewer stories; more decisions.

Because you'll ask for an example you can hold up against a calendar, here's how a tidy month inside a build might feel for a triathlete heading towards a 70.3, described without a spreadsheet. Week one opens with a sweet-spot bike you finish with something left, a threshold run that feels like breathing hard without bargaining, and a swim where the catch finally stays connected across the last 200s. The long ride at the weekend holds a steady block where fuelling is on time and the brick jog that follows is quiet and short enough to make you smile. Week two leans into cadence and posture on the bike and a long run that settles before it asks for a few minutes at race feel. The swim is mechanics into steady rather than drama into pride. Midweek you slide in a short brick because your calendar allows, not because you're trying to be interesting. Week three puts teeth back in: a bike session that revisits sweet-spot with one extra rep, a run that stitches together four tidy threshold blocks, and an open-water swim where you practise starts and settling without the nervous theatre. You ride long again, this time a touch further, and you eat early, because you said you would. Week four loosens: twenty-five per cent less volume across the board, one short taste of threshold so your legs remember, more sleep, fewer late nights with your phone. You exit the month looking forward to the next one. That's the signal the plan is working.

If you're a runner in late base rather than a triathlete in build, the same paragraph reads differently but feels the same: you finish easy runs with more in the tank; your weekly threshold set remains civilised; your long run alternates between purely easy and gently progressive; you stride twice a week and feel quicker without feeling brave; you strength train twice and stop before you chase soreness; you sleep enough times to feel proud.

It's easy to overcomplicate gear when seasons get serious. Keep equipment simple and serviceable. Fresh tyres and sensible pressures do more for your bike split than another carbon bolt. Shoes that still have midsole life do more for your long run than a fourth pair that lives in the box. A wetsuit pulled properly into your armpits and hips changes more about your swim than a new model you wear wrong. Fit that you can hold for an hour does more than a position you can hold for a photo. Buy simplicity that gets used. Ignore complexity that makes you feel fast on the internet. The season is not a catalogue; it's a sequence of days you can actually do.

Nutrition belongs to the season as much as to the session. In base, you're establishing habits: regular meals, enough carbohydrates to support the work, protein spread across the day. In build, you practise race-like intakes inside long sessions so your gut learns the job before the number pin appears. In peak, you confirm rather than experiment. Race week pasta isn't a religion; it's a reminder that glycogen matters and that your stomach likes familiar food under stress. Post-race you eat what sounds like kindness. There is nothing to prove at the dinner table.

A few places people consistently come unstuck, and a sentence to steer each one. Too many big races too close together: choose one to serve and one to learn. No reset week: schedule it now while you feel good. A build that never ends: make recovery weeks automatic. Peaking by panic: sharpen, don't search. Treating every group session like a referendum on your fitness: keep one for fun and let the rest serve the plan. Calling a deload "lazy": it's how you cash the cheque.

If you like an actionable end to a chapter, here's yours. Pick up your calendar. Mark the A-race. Ring the two weeks after it as "Reset" and protect them from your enthusiastic future self. Count back: give yourself two or three weeks to peak, eight to twelve to build, six to ten to lay base, and two to four at the start to breathe. Label one or two B-races you'll use to learn. Write one line for each of the next four weeks—no poetry, just purpose: "Base: frequency + strength." "Base: skills first." "Build: threshold clarity." "Build: brick rhythm." Put the lighter week in ink. On a sticky note, write the rule you'll follow when life hits: defend one quality session and one long; everything else floats. Put it where you'll see it.

Your season won't be perfect. It doesn't need to be. It should sound like your life and feel like a story you want to live: steady start, focused middle, sharp finish, honest exhale. Build it that way and you'll stop guessing week to week and start arriving when it counts.

Chapter 10 – Recovery, Real Life & Training That Sticks

If training is the engine, recovery is the oil. Ignore it long enough and the whole thing starts to grind. Not in a dramatic, cinematic way—just a slow squeak that turns into a drag you try to outrun with more effort. That's the maddening part: when you're tired, working harder looks like an answer. Most of the time, it's the cul-de-sac.

And yes, most "recovery" advice reads like it was written for people with two naps a day, a massage table in the spare room, and no unread emails. This chapter is for the rest of us: the ones who train in between meetings and school runs, who fall asleep on the sofa with wet hair after a late swim, who have good weeks, strange weeks, and weeks that are basically admin in running shoes. You don't need more rituals. You need a system that notices you're human—and still delivers.

This is how we make recovery part of training, not a guilty afterthought. It's how you adapt sessions to the week you're living, not the week you imagined. It's how you hold a plan lightly enough that it doesn't snap at the first sign of real life.

Let's start with the part most people resist: recovery isn't a prize you earn by being perfect. It's a condition of entry. Without it, your body adapts less and complains more. You've seen it—fitness flattens even though you're "working." Sleep frays. Mood goes thin. Easy paces creep upward while the heart rate won't come down. Little pains start arriving in patterns so regular you could set a watch by them. That's not weakness; that's information. You're not fragile. You're under-recovered.

Recovery has boring jobs that keep you interesting. It repairs muscle tissue you stressed on purpose. It refuels glycogen so tomorrow's session is about your engine, not your empty tank. It steadies the nervous system so "hard" is a choice, not your default. It keeps the immune system from tapping out just as your build hits its stride. The adaptation you want from training happens when you're not training. It's wild how many athletes know that and still argue with it.

The fix is not to chase perfection. It's to make recovery automatic in small ways every day, visible every week, planned every few weeks, and flexible when life swings. That's the whole brief.

Daily first, because that's where the foundation sits. Sleep is the quiet king here. Not a magical number—just enough, often enough, to let the work count. In practice that means going to bed fifteen minutes earlier than you currently do and protecting two nights a week like they're sessions. It means cutting the scrolling that makes you tired while doing nothing to make you sleepy. It means understanding that one late night doesn't ruin a training block—but two or three stacked will change how every session feels.

Nutrition is the other daily lever with the biggest swing. You don't need a spreadsheet. You do need to eat enough, on time, and in a way that respects the training you've chosen. If you're someone who "forgets" to eat because the morning got away from you, fix the environment before you fix yourself: stash something practical where you work; put a bottle where your eyes fall; decide your post-session meal before you start the session so the decision doesn't collide with fatigue. If you regularly finish hard work under-fuelled, you're teaching your body to treat stress as scarcity. That lesson shows up as flat sessions and a brain that believes "training is hard" when training is actually underfed.

Breath and mobility are not personality traits. They're tools. Five minutes of nose-led breathing down on the floor after a noisy day tilts your nervous system back toward "I can absorb this." Two minutes of ankle work before a run or shoulder-blade work before a swim takes less time than your watch looking for GPS and changes how your tissues feel on the other side. We're not trying to reinvent you. We're trying to lower the friction at the parts of the day where most people blink and lose twenty minutes to nothing.

Coach's note: if a recovery habit needs a new personality to sustain it, it's the wrong habit. Shrink it until you'll actually do it.

Weekly next, because rhythm beats heroics. A good week has a shape you can recognise: hard days that actually ask, easy days that actually restore, and one day where training doesn't exist on the page at all. You don't earn that rest day. You schedule it because the next week deserves it. The easy sessions aren't punishment. They're how you arrive ready for the sessions that change you.

When people tell me they don't "feel" their easy days, that's the point. You're not supposed to. Easy is circulation, tissue health, and headspace. It's where you hold posture without cost. It's where you practise the skill of keeping easy truly easy so your body understands the difference between stress and support. Most consistency is built on that distinction.

And if you're thinking, "But my life is already full," then we're speaking the same language. Smart weeks contain flex by design. You defend one quality session and one long session that suit your phase. Everything else can move or shrink without theatre. That's not laziness. That's architecture.

Zoom out again. Blocks need recovery, too. Every third or fourth week, your plan should loosen. Not because you've failed to keep up, but because you've succeeded in applying consistent stress and now you're making space to absorb it. Volume drops. The hardest work trims back to a taste, so speed and rhythm don't vanish. You sleep more because you can and also because you choose to. You review the last few weeks with a two-line debrief after each key session— how it felt, what you learned—so the next block starts with eyes open. It's not a holiday from training. It's how you cash the cheque.

Connor didn't believe that. He was the rhythm of a thousand spreadsheets: consistent, driven, allergic to stepping back. Week seven of every build, he'd hit a wall. We didn't add supplements or lectures. We did three plain things. We put a recovery week in ink every fourth week. We moved his alarms so 5 a.m. sessions didn't happen after abbreviated nights. We added two short sessions he couldn't argue with: breath and mobility on days where his mind told him to "do something." Eight weeks in, his quality sessions stuck. His long rides didn't ruin the week. He stopped using rest as a test of character. He didn't get weaker. He got faster because he finally let the work count.

Real life arrives on its own schedule. Pretending otherwise is how you end up resenting training for being brittle. So we write plans that survive normal chaos. The logic is simple. Every week has anchors and floats. Anchors are the sessions that define the week in your current phase— maybe that's the Tuesday threshold run and the Saturday long ride. Floats are the sessions that add polish but can move or vanish without guilt. When life swings, you defend the anchors and let the floats go. No speeches. No starting again Monday. You're still in your season. You're just steering.

Sometimes, life doesn't swing. It punches. You miss a week. Or two. You got sick. Your child didn't sleep for a fortnight. Work set itself on fire. Breathe. Missing days is not the problem; panic is. Don't cram. Don't try to be the person you were three weeks ago by Wednesday. Pick up where you are, not where the calendar says you should be. Scale volume for a few days. Keep intensity as controlled tastes rather than meals. Restart with a small win you can bank—thirty minutes easy, one short quality touch, ten minutes of strength with shapes you own. Fitness is cumulative. It's hard to destroy and easy to mute. Calm re-entry is how you find it again.

Coach's note: the habit you keep beats the session you chase.

Illness has its own rules. Above the neck and mild? Light work might be fine. Below the neck, fever, or the kind of fatigue that makes stairs feel like intervals. You rest. After fever, give yourself forty-eight quiet hours and return at sixty to seventy percent for a few days. It will feel too slow. You'll be tempted to hurry. That temptation is how people start the same cold twice.

Injury niggles are more like whispers than alarms. They do you a favour by repeating themselves. If the same tendon speaks at the same point in the same session every week, it's not cursing you. It's handing you the lesson: the dose is wrong or the pattern is. Change the surface. Trim the rep length. Split the long session into two shorter ones. Swap paddles for a pull buoy and focus on catch positions without tugging your shoulder through glue. Trade one run for one bike for ten days and keep your identity intact while the tissue calms. You're not fragile. You're adaptable.

Because this is real life, let's talk shifts, travel, and stress that doesn't show on your watch. If you work nights or rotate, your training responds to sleep, not the clock. The day after a long night is not for threshold. It's for easy circulation, a nap if it's on the table, and food that's more than coffee. Put quality on days when your sleep resembles sleep. If you travel, protect two sessions: one quality touch and one longer aerobic session. Hotel gyms can hold your positions with fifteen minutes of carries, hinges, and light pulls. Your suitcase can hold a band for shoulder-blade work. If you're in an airport on what the plan calls "threshold day," the plan is wrong. The athlete is right there, living. Adjust.

Stress is elastic. Sometimes it's the training that needs to flex. If work is on fire and your brain feels like a browser with fifty tabs open, your threshold session is not a place to prove you can still do everything. Use the same structure, cut one rep, widen the recoveries, and insist on even effort. You'll get ninety percent of the adaptation for half the cost. Or move the session entirely and choose a long walk in daylight. Not because walking is magic, but because you're not a robot and nervous systems don't live in spreadsheets.

You can train recovery as a skill. People hate hearing that because it sounds like extra work. It isn't. It's noticing earlier, deciding sooner, and shrinking the interruption.

Noticing earlier looks like this: you realise you're bargaining with the session before you've even put your shoes on; you see easy paces finally stop drifting up after a deload; you catch yourself snapping at someone you love for something that doesn't matter and recognise it as a training symptom, not a personality flaw. Deciding sooner looks like this: you scale a session at the first sign of ugly form; you stop a rep short when you feel your posture collapsing; you swap the second coffee for water and an apple because your head is fizzy and your body is asking for anything but more of the same. Shrinking the interruption looks like this: you build a micro warm-down habit—two minutes of easy and a long exhale—so your body stops buzzing before you slam into the next thing.

None of that is glamorous. All of it adds up.

People ask for gadgets here. Wearables are fine if you own the narrative. If your recovery score is a number that helps you choose sleep, great. If it's a number that tells you your day before your day begins, bin it. Your notes are better data. Two lines after key sessions—feel and lesson—teach you what your tech is trying to hint at. Over a month, patterns show. That's the only timescale that matters for real training.

If you like rules, have just a few. If you sleep fewer than six and a half hours for two nights in a row, the next day is not for quality unless the season absolutely demands it and you absolutely know you can handle it. If your heart rate sits ten beats high on an easy run and it isn't heat, caffeine, or a hill, you slow down and finish easy, or you finish early. If the same niggle repeats on the same day, the next week changes. If you're ill, you rest without bargaining. If you missed a week, you don't make it up; you return scaled.

Coach's note: recovery conversations are clear when they're written before the week, not invented after you're tired.

What does a recovery-smart week feel like when it's working? Strangely normal. You go to bed on purpose twice. You start two sessions slower than you felt like starting and finish them feeling clever for it. You place your easiest day next to your longest, not out of guilt but out of design. You eat before you're hungry once. You cancel a social ride because it's going to turn into a mid-week race and you want your Saturday legs. You do a twenty-minute mobility and breath session while the pasta boils. Your watch thinks you were boring. Your body thinks you were kind. The following week thanks you by letting you do what you actually planned.

If the week goes sideways, the plan doesn't need drama. You lop the garnish off the top. Defend one quality and one long. If both are impossible, choose the one that keeps your identity intact. For most, that's the long—time on feet or time in the saddle is where confidence lives. Next week, you return to normal, not to penance.

The hardest part of recovery isn't a behaviour. It's guilt. You've been taught that rest feels like an excuse. You've been praised for grinding. So when you back off, your head tells you stories about losing your edge. The fastest way to quiet those stories is evidence. Keep a simple ledger once a week for eight weeks: sessions started on time; nights you slept like it mattered; times you scaled without sulking; instances you fuelled before you faded; one decision you made that won't show up on Strava but changed your day. You're not doing this to feel good about yourself. You're doing it because brains are bad historians and good prosecutors. Give yours a record worth defending.

This is where recovery, real life, and training that sticks tie together: you make room. Not theoretical room—actual space in your week where nothing happens on purpose. You build your plan with exits that don't feel like failure.

You accept that the most "productive" day occasionally looks like not training. You learn the difference between "tired because I trained" and "tired because I'm alive," and you treat them differently. You stop waiting for motivation and start relying on systems that still work when you're not in the mood.

In practice, that looks like a family calendar that knows about your long ride and your partner's long morning. It looks like setting your kit the night before not because you're disciplined, but because future-you is chaotic and deserves help. It looks like adding five minutes of floor work to the end of your day when your brain says there's no time, and discovering there was always five minutes; it was just hiding under your phone.

It also looks like joy. Recovery isn't dour. It's the absence of dread. It's the return of appetite—for training, for racing, for the feeling that you're building something. You can't grind your way into that. You build it by not emptying the jar every time you feel brave.

If you only keep a handful of lines from this chapter, keep these. Recovery isn't earned. It's required. Missed sessions don't derail you; panic does. Rest isn't a sign you're soft; it's a sign you're serious. Easy means easy—on purpose, not by accident. Sleep is training. Food is training. Breath is training. Scaling is a skill. The long game is the only game worth playing.

Pause & apply, because theory without an action is another paragraph you nod at and forget. Choose two nights this week you'll defend sleep. Choose one session you'll start slower than you want and finish proud. Put one simple meal plan next to one hard session. Write your two-line debrief after your next quality day. Schedule one day with no training at all and don't replace it with guilt. If you miss a session, don't negotiate with the calendar; carry on scaled. And if a niggle speaks twice, change something the third time.

Your body adapts in space. Your confidence grows in space. Make space part of your system and you'll stop surviving blocks—you'll start finishing them with room to grow. That's training that sticks. That's a season that lasts.

Chapter 11 – Race Day: Confidence, Chaos & Getting It Right When It Counts

Race day is never just racing day. It's the sum of all the ordinary sessions you stacked, the early alarms you didn't want, the choices you made when nobody was looking. It's nerves and hope and a bag of kit that suddenly feels like a riddle. It's family on the barrier, a number on your chest, the quiet thought you don't say out loud: I hope today shows the work. And yes—there's always a bit of chaos. That's why we plan for it calmly and in advance, so when the noise arrives you can do the simple things well.

This chapter is a reality check and a rehearsal. Not just how to pace, but how to feel ready. How to manage the hours before the gun. How to make decisions when your watch, the weather, or your stomach has its own ideas. The goal isn't a perfect day. It's your day—executed with enough composure that your fitness can speak.

Race day doesn't only test fitness. It tests routine—can you do what you said you'd do under pressure? It tests nutrition—does your plan survive real appetite, real heat, real nerves? It tests resilience—how quickly do you return to the task after something small goes sideways? It tests emotion—can you keep your effort choices steady when the start feels like a sprint and the middle feels like a verdict? Above all, it tests belief, because you'll have to choose your own plan over someone else's pace more than once.

The plan is not a guarantee. It's a set of anchors you can hold when everything else tries to drag you around. We don't chase certainty—we build options. That's the shape of race-day readiness.

There are three parts to being ready, and they overlap. Physical readiness means your body has already met the intensity you'll ask of it and knows how it feels when you're a little tired. Mental readiness means you've rehearsed how to handle the short stretch from okay to uncomfortable without arguing with it. Logistical readiness means you've tested the kit, the food, and the transitions you'll use; you know what bag each item lives in and where it goes next. No voodoo. Just boring things done in a way that survives noise.

Alex is a good example of how small things add up. He texted the night before a target race: I don't think I've done enough. He had. The feeling wasn't data; it was nerves. We pointed him back to his own log and asked him to read the last eight weeks, not the last eight minutes. We walked through the plan—efforts, intake, cues—and then sent him to bed with a simple breathing drill: slow, long exhales to leave the phone alone and let the body shut down. He didn't wake up fearless. He woke up with a job. He ran a negative split and set a PB. The fitness mattered. The system let it show.

Race week is a taper in miniature—shorter, tidier, steadier. Keep frequency. Trim volume. Keep brief tastes of race feel so rhythm stays close. The week works if it feels almost boring. One day early in the week you touch the pace you'll hold, but only in short bites. One day you rehearse logistics in a light brick or a quick transition run, not to make yourself tired but to remind your body where everything goes. One or two days you do easy work with a few strides so your legs don't feel neglected. One day you are genuinely off your feet because rest is part of readiness. You pack earlier than you think. You eat what you know. You picture the first five minutes and the last five—and leave the middle to the process.

If the race is on a Sunday, that might look like this in feel, not just in boxes: Monday you move easily and let stiffness drain. Tuesday you sharpen—four short efforts at race feel with plenty of easy between. Wednesday you downshift and do the little things. Thursday you do a brief rehearsal—bike and a calm run off it, or a short race-pace segment on the run—then call it. Friday you pack, stretch, and stop inventing changes. Saturday you travel or shake out, ten to twenty minutes with a few strides, done before you can start measuring yourself against strangers. Sunday you wake with a plan you've already used in your head.

Race morning is mostly logistics. You get up early enough to eat without rushing. You eat the same kind of breakfast you've used in long sessions—something your stomach recognises. You drink some fluid and stop before you slosh. You get to the venue with more minutes than you need because time is the cheapest calm. You set your space—bike racked cleanly, shoes where your hands will find them, numbers and nutrition where you don't have to think. You check your tyres without turning it into a ritual. You get in the queue for the bathroom and you stay friendly, because nerves are contagious and so is calm.

If you're swimming first, you stand on the shore and take three long exhales. You pull your suit high—armpits and hips—so your shoulders can move. You sight a line. You decide to start a shade easier than your ego wants because everyone else will do the opposite. If you're starting a run race, you agree with yourself that the first kilometre will be deliberately boring. If you're cycling first in a TT, you look at the first ten minutes on your head unit and decide to make them the steadiest you do all day.

Everything you do that morning should be a copy of something you've done before. Race day is not the day for a new gel, a different sock, or a brand-new lacing trick. Old, known, simple—that's the lane.

Pacing is a choice you make more than once. It's not set by the number you saw on a Sunday three weeks ago. It's anchored by it, then adjusted for the day. If it's hot, the numbers are slower at the same effort—no verdict, just physiology. If it's windy, you protect effort and position rather than trying to impress yourself up a false flat. If the course rolls, you let pace drift on climbs and hold effort, then you carry speed on the other side. If you're running, you let heart rate climb slowly through the first third rather than sprinting to your threshold and then trying to hold the line with grit.

You can keep your cues short. "Even, even, strong" works for a half marathon. "Quiet hands, long exhale" works for the opening of a swim. "Cadence is control" works for bike segments that punish grinders. The trick is to choose cues you actually hear when your head gets loud. That usually means fewer words, not more.

Nutrition is the other half of pacing. You start early because waiting until you're hungry or flat is a trap. You sip regularly on the bike because that's where intake is easiest, and you don't try to make the run fix what the bike forgot. You carry what you've trained with. If the course offers something you didn't, you treat it as a bonus, not a solution. If your stomach turns against you, you slow a little, you choose a simpler intake for a few minutes, and you let the gut catch up. Panic is the enemy; calm is a strategy.

Transitions turn deliberate days into messy ones when people try to win the race in a car park. You don't. You move like a person who knows the order. After the swim you walk the first few metres if the world is spinning so your heart rate remembers it's attached to a body. You get out of the suit without a wrestling match because you've practised it. You get on the bike without proving anything in the first minute. You get off the bike with feet that know how to be feet again because you've practised short off-bike jogs at calm pace.

If you're running only, the "transition" is the first kilometre. Make it dull. Let your cadence settle. Let your breathing find its slot. The time you "save" by rushing the first five minutes is the time you pay back—with interest—when you're ten kilometres in and wishing you could start again.

Races have personalities. Heat asks for patience and fluid. Cold asks for hands that can still function—zipper, gels, bottles—so you wear enough to keep control rather than pretending you're immune. Rain asks for calm feet and extra space in corners. Wind asks for posture before ego. Crowds ask you to hold your line and your plan. Early surges from other people ask you to say no without saying anything. Your job is not to stop the weather or the field. Your job is to stay with your own decisions.

Tech has its own personality. Sometimes it sulks. Watches decide to freeze; power metres won't pair; a strap reads a heart rate for a hummingbird. If the numbers die, your plan shouldn't. You've practised the feel of the pace you want, the sound of your breathing when it's right, the way your strides fall at race cadence. You're not a hostage to a screen. If a device fails, you choose effort and you go. If later the file is useless, the race is not. You weren't racing your computer.

The middle of the race is where people go looking for meaning. It's just where work lives. You don't need heroics there. You need repetition. Drink when you said you would. Stay tall when you'd like to fold. Remind your shoulders they're not part of your legs. If you feel great, you don't cash it all right away. If you feel average, you don't drag a story into it. If you feel rough, you don't assume it's permanent. You change one thing—cadence up five beats, sip now, shake the arms out—and you give it five minutes. The number of problems solved by changing one thing for five minutes is higher than you think.

Trouble comes in a few predictable costumes. Cramps? Often a pacing or position issue more than a salt mystery. Ease slightly, adjust cadence, take on fluid, relax the jaw and shoulders. Side stitch? Exhale longer on the opposite side for a few breaths, slow a fraction, then return. Panic in the water? Roll to the side, long exhale, a few strokes of breaststroke or heads-up freestyle to sight and settle, then back to rhythm. GI revolt? Stop the war. Slow a little, choose water, then reintroduce carbs in small sips. Most crises are loud for a short time and quiet if you don't feed them drama.

Late race is where you go from protecting your day to expressing your work. If you've kept the middle honest, the last third is where "strong" can show up. The best version of strong usually looks less like a sprint and more like not slowing down while everyone else does. That's still heroism. It just doesn't look noisy.

If your plan included negative splits, the ask is simple: stop slowing. If your plan included a final segment at set effort, you hold it there rather than hunting for numbers you liked in training. You'll see people around you paying bills they wrote in the first half. You don't need to collect them. You just need to keep the line you've been drawing.

When you cross the line, your body still needs a coach. That's you. You walk. You drink something that isn't a performance of toughness. You eat something your stomach recognises. If you're dizzy, you sit with your knees up and breathe until the world stops tilting. You resist the immediate urge to sign up for another race because feelings are loud and calendars are quiet. You let the moment be a moment.

Reflection is how the day becomes useful. Not an essay—just honest notes before memory flatters or erases. What went well? Where did you keep your head? What did you learn about pace on this course? What did your stomach say about timing? What will you do the same? What will you do differently—and how will you practise that difference? There are no points for poetry. The value is in sentences you'll believe when you read them next time.

Then you reset. That might be a few days if the race was short. It might be a week or two if it was long. You're not losing fitness. You're consolidating it. This is where the next chapter begins, even if you aren't writing it yet.

Because triathlon has more moving parts, let's be clear without turning this into a checklist you'll forget. The swim starts calmer than your heart wants. You breathe early and often. You sight enough to stay honest but not so much you swim like a meerkat. You find feet that match your effort and you sit there without tapping. You turn buoys wider than the scrum. You exit the water with deliberate steps and make your hands useful before your legs pretend they're already on the bike.

The bike opens steady. You don't go chasing numbers you liked in cool air on a flat Tuesday. You eat early. You drink earlier. You keep your posture when the course insists on headwinds. You hold your line politely. You don't follow a surge you didn't author. You get off the bike with legs that know the cadence they'll use in the first kilometre.

The run opens quiet. Your watch is not a judge in the first kilometre; it's a reference, later. You choose cues you can hear: tall, calm, easy breath, quick feet. You take fluid at the first station even if you think you don't need it. You build by feel, not by impulse. You stop looking for signs and you start making them—every time you hold form past a corner, every time you take an aid station smoothly, every time you bring attention back to the task after the brain wanders. If the day is good, you don't empty the tank at halfway. If the day is average, you stay with it. If the day is rough, you do small good things and let time do its job. It's surprising how often "rough" turns into "fine" if you give it ten minutes of sensible choices.

For a road race, the themes are the same, just fewer moving parts. The start is crowded and full of lies. You'll feel too fast at an easy pace; you'll feel obliged to match the flow. You don't. First kilometre boring, then build. Your first ten minutes are for locating rhythm, not proving anything. Middle segments are where you commit to even effort and keep your food and water plan honest. The last third is for control: hold shape, hold cadence, hold decisions. If you're chasing a time, don't do arithmetic that spirals you out of the race. Split the distance into manageable strips: to the next turn, to the next landmark, to the next station. The faster runner at your level is almost always the steadier one.

Shoes you've worn. Socks that don't experiment. Laces you've checked. Breakfast that isn't a prank. A hat or glasses if sun or showers are in play. Documented start corral time that includes the bathroom queue you always underestimate. That's "logistics." It's not glamorous, but it's what makes the day feel like you've done this before— because you have, in smaller pieces.

Confidence on race day is not loud. It's quiet evidence you can point at: sessions done, paces felt, skills rehearsed, mornings managed. Loud confidence tries to drown out doubt with noise and often spends itself early. Quiet confidence stands on choices you can repeat. If you need a single sentence to carry with you, make it literal and plain. Strong legs, calm head. Even now, even here. One effort at a time. It doesn't need to inspire you. It needs to direct you.

If nerves spike, you shrink the task. Bring it back to what you control in the next five minutes: breathe out longer than you breathe in; drop your shoulders; drink on schedule; keep your cadence; run the line you picked; ride the power you chose; swim the stroke you know. When the noise fades, the plan is still there waiting.

A final note, because this is the part most people miss while chasing better training. Race day is not an exam you pass. It's a chance to express work you've already done. If you anchor to that, you'll handle the chaos without turning it into a story about who you are. You'll make decisions because they're useful, not because they prove anything.

You'll leave with a result, yes—but more importantly, you'll leave with a process you can repeat.

Take that process into the next start line and the next. You're not looking for magic. You're building a day you can trust. That's how confidence shows up when it counts. That's how chaos turns into something you can ride. That's how your race becomes yours.

Chapter 12 – Reflect, Reset & Repeat: The Loop That Builds Lifelong Athletes

The race is done. Medal on a ribbon. Salt on your skin. Someone shoves a banana into your hand and the world feels oddly quiet even though a speaker is still shouting names. You've showered, eaten everything in sight, and maybe cried a bit in the car on the way home. Now what?

This is the part nobody really prepares you for—the after. Pride and fatigue show up together. Restlessness taps your shoulder. Your legs are tired; your brain is loud. A part of you wants to enter three more races before the endorphins fade. Another part wonders what to do with your body tomorrow morning at 6 a.m., when habit tries to drag you out of bed. Wherever you are on that spectrum, pause. Not because you need to stop. Because this moment matters.

This is where reflection happens. This is where lessons settle. This is where athletes either grow—or simply repeat the same season with a new number pinned on. Before you buy another entry, before you open a new spreadsheet, take stock. What worked? What didn't? What surprised you? What did you learn about yourself—not just on the day, but in the weeks and months it took to get there?

Medals are nice. The story you can tell yourself with a straight face—that's the win that lasts.

Reflection isn't wallowing and it isn't a forensic audit. It's a short, honest conversation that turns experience into fuel. Most people skip it. They move on too quickly ("What's next?") or they spiral into analysis that makes training feel like homework. The middle ground is where progress lives: capture what mattered while the detail is still warm, then move.

Start simple. Three short notes within forty-eight hours of finishing: what went well; what was harder than expected; what you'll do the same or differently next time. No essays. No speeches. The point is to anchor memory before your brain edits the day into a tidy legend or a disaster movie. This is also the moment to notice what changed in you that doesn't show on a watch: you started your long sessions without negotiating, you learned to back off a rep before form broke, you stopped turning every easy day into a quiet race. Those lines are harder to capture than splits, and they're more valuable.

If writing is painful, voice-note it on a walk. If you don't want to look at your file yet, don't. Facts will still be there tomorrow. The feeling won't. Record that first.

Coach's note: reflection is most useful when it sounds like you on a tired evening, not a press release after a win.

A race tests more than your fitness. It tests your systems. Routine under pressure. Nutrition when nerves are real, not theoretical. The way you handle a watch that won't behave, a crowd that runs your first kilometre for you, a wind that rearranges your plan. When things unravel—and something always will—you fall back on what you've practised. That's why we rehearse starts, transitions, cues, fuelling. But the post-race loop matters just as much. Reflect. Reset. Repeat. The athletes who do this cleanly don't just get better times; they build better seasons.

Emily is the neat version of the lesson. She knocked seven minutes off her 10K and felt bulletproof for an hour and empty after dinner. At 10 p.m. she sent a link: another race the next weekend. We paused instead. Walked through her notes. She didn't need another start line. She needed a week where her legs caught up and her head did, too. On paper her biggest gain was the time. In practice it was the change underneath: her pacing cues worked, her mid-race "don't chase" decision held, and she didn't turn a wobble at kilometre seven into a story about failure. She took a gentle reset, then built back to a second 10K ten weeks later and ran faster again with less noise. The difference wasn't fitness. It was the loop.

Not every after looks like Emily's. Sometimes the day collapses. You miss a target by a lot. You DNF. You pick up a niggle. The temptation is to sprint away from the feeling or to make it permanent. Neither helps. A bad day doesn't void good training. It just sends you a clear invoice. Before you pay it with ego, ask better questions. Did the conditions legitimately change the day? Did you stick to your eating, or did you forget until the wheels went? Was your pacing built for the course you ran or the one you hoped you'd see? Did your sleep in the last week look like something a human could race from? None of those lines are excuses. They're the levers you can pull.

Make space for disappointment without turning it into identity. Tell one person you trust the unedited version. Then do the same three notes: what went well (there was something); what was harder than expected (be precise); what you'll change (one or two things, not twelve). When the sting fades, you'll be glad you left breadcrumbs for yourself.

Reset is the part people try to bargain with. They cut it short because they're excited or they extend it until training feels unfamiliar again. The middle is the move. After big efforts, a short physical and mental reset is not soft. It's strategic.

Physically, you drop intensity. You move easily. You choose surfaces and sessions that feel like circulation, not proof. Walk. Swim steady. Spin on the turbo with a podcast. Do twenty minutes of mobility because you always say you will and then don't. Sleep a little more. Eat like a human being, not a spreadsheet. None of this deletes fitness. It consolidates it.

Mentally, you take the pressure off. You let yourself like training again before you ask it to be important. You text a training partner about coffee without suggesting a threshold set. You write two lines a day for a week: what felt good; what felt off. You let your head catch up with your legs.

Planning-wise, you keep it small. No grand declarations. One focus for the next four weeks written in plain language you can't misunderstand: consistency plus strength; skills first; threshold clarity; brick rhythm. Reset isn't the space for setting six goals. It's the space for finding your feet again.

How long? Shorter than your anxiety and longer than your ego. After a 5K, three to five days often does it. After a half marathon or 70.3, seven to ten days. After a marathon or

Ironman, ten to fourteen before you pretend you're a sprightly deer again. If you come back early and feel flat, you're not broken—you're early. Step back one more day. It's fine.

Coach's note: if you want to shorten reset because you "feel amazing," keep one easy day in the bank. Spend it when the buzz fades.

If reflection is the what, and reset is the space, repeat is the craft. You start again—not from scratch, from experience. The next block is not a new you. It's the same you with better notes, sharper boundaries, and a clearer sense of what matters.

Bring forward the few things that actually changed your training. Maybe it was staging your kit the night before because mornings are chaos. Maybe it was holding easy pace on easy days even when group chat pulled the other way. Maybe it was adding a five-minute warm-up for your shoulders before you got in the water. Keep the tiny things that bought you disproportionate calm.

Leave behind the things that made you feel busy but didn't move the line. If your week turned into a scavenger hunt for five different metrics and you felt clever but tired, pick two. If a watch score dictated your mood more than your notes did, put the device on "quiet" for a while. If you ran hard because your friend did and then paid for it for three days, keep one social session for fun and make the others serve the plan. Simpler sticks.

The repeat loop also needs a guardrail: the week you miss is not the week you repay. If travel, illness, or life pulls a thread, you don't cram. You pick up where you are, scaled for a few days, then resume the plan. That habit alone will save more seasons than a new pair of shoes.

You can make this practical without turning it into homework. After every A-race—or at the end of any block you care about—create two short things: a debrief you'll actually read and a one-page next block.

The debrief is a single page, divided into four quarters. Top left: what went well (training habits, race choices, one or two numbers that matter). Top right: what was harder than expected (be factual, not dramatic). Bottom left: what you'll repeat (behaviours, not just sessions). Bottom right: what you'll change (no more than three). Date it. File it where you can find it when your next taper gets noisy.

The one-page next block answers five questions in boring language: what's the focus; what are the weekly anchors; what's the minimum viable week when life swings; what are two cues you'll use in sessions; what's your rule for sleep. Put it somewhere you'll see it. The purpose isn't inspiration. It's direction.

There's another piece to the loop that doesn't get discussed because it feels unsexy: the blues. Post-race dips are common. You spend months pointing at a thing and then the thing is gone and your calendar looks like an empty room. That emptiness can feel like freedom or like a hole. Neither is permanent. The cure isn't signing up for something else in a panic. The cure is doing small normal things on purpose. Choose one easy session that reminds your body what rhythm feels like. Choose one short social thing that isn't a race. Choose one non-training task you've ignored that the rest of your life will appreciate. Momentum returns faster when you stop asking it to knock.

Social media can make the blues louder. People post their best days; your brain compares them to your worst. The way out is to narrow your field of view. Share your reflection with one or two people who understand the project. Resist the recap if you're prone to perform it. Quiet is a training aid. You can return to the noise when you're not listening for your own voice.

A few patterns repeat every season, and how you handle them decides whether you become the steady person you keep saying you want to be.

The first is the rebound. You had a good day and you feel invincible. Or you had a bad day and you want a rematch. Either way, your finger is hovering over the sign-up button. The counter-move isn't "never sign up." It's "not yet." Sleep two nights. Write your three notes. Do a short reset. If you still want it on Wednesday with the same clarity you had on Sunday, by all means. You'll be doing it for a reason, not a feeling.

The second is the rewrite. You decide, after a race, to be a completely new athlete: more volume, more intensity, more everything. It reads well in your head. In practice, it breaks. Keep one change per block. Earn the right to add more by showing you can live with one.

The third is the exile. The race didn't go to plan, so you disappear until you feel "worthy" again. Training isn't a courtroom. It's a craft. You don't need to be worthy to work. You need to work to remember why you like it. Return quietly. Let small wins rebuild your appetite.

Coach's note: the person who learns fastest isn't the one who hurts the most—it's the one who observes the most.

Because triathlon has more moving parts, the loop can feel busier. It doesn't need to be. The same rhythm works. For multisport, your first forty-eight hours are about body care (hydrate, eat, light movement), equipment sanity (wash, check, store), and the brief note you'll thank yourself for later. Your reset week looks like three or four low-stress sessions with a bias toward swimming and easy spins because feet and tendons love you more when you're kind on ground. Your repeat begins with skills before load: water timing, bike posture, run cadence. Then the teeth come back.

Runners can do similar, scaled by distance. After a marathon, accept that the body and head need longer than a half. After a 5K or 10K, your return is quicker, but the need for a pause doesn't vanish. The loop is about respect, not distance.

Strength belongs to the after as much as the before. In the reset you hold shapes—hinge, split squat, row—with light loads and full control. In the repeat you rebuild intention— slower eccentrics, cleaner positions, one rep in the tank. That alone makes your next build feel smoother.

Nutrition sits in both spaces. Post-race, eat like recovery is a thing. In reset, eat to rebuild—not to compensate for what you think you did or didn't earn on the course. In repeat, go back to the basics that worked in training: consistent meals, enough carbohydrate for the work, protein across the day, and the fuel you'll use again next time practised inside sessions, not guessed at on race week.

Sleep stitches the whole loop together. Two protected nights in the first four after a race will do more for your body than a bag of tricks. Two protected nights in the first week of a new block will do more for your consistency than a new device. You know this. Write it down anyway.

If you like tidy endings with something to do, here's yours.

Tonight, write three lines about your last block or race: what went well; what was harder than expected; what you'll keep or change. Put a date on it. Then schedule your reset: the number of days you'll keep intensity away, the number of easy sessions you'll allow, the time you'll go to bed twice this week because future-you always finds a reason to stay up. Then draft your one-page next block in plain language: focus, anchors, minimum viable week, two cues, sleep rule. That's it. No graphics. No fantasy miles. Paper beats mood.

If you only keep a handful of sentences from this chapter, keep these. Training doesn't end at the finish line. That's where it begins again. Smart athletes reflect—not to dwell, but to grow. Reset isn't a reward; it's how you bank your work. Progress is a loop. Embrace it. You don't need to be perfect. You need to be consistent, curious, and willing to start again with small, good decisions.

And if you're still here, reading—good. That means you care about more than one day. Reset. Reflect. Repeat. You're just getting started.

Chapter 13 – The Mental Game: Grit, Focus & Fire When It Counts

Here's the truth most athletes discover the hard way: you can be the fittest person on the start line and still come apart in the middle. Not because your legs forgot how to move, but because your head forgot how to help. Performance is physical, yes—but it's also attention, emotion, choice. The mental game isn't about pretending you're fearless. It's about staying useful when fear shows up anyway.

You don't need slogans. You need habits you can use at 4 a.m. on race morning and at minute 37 when the plan gets noisy. You need a way to steer your thoughts without wrestling them, to hold effort when your brain suggests a detour, to believe in yourself on days when recent results would argue otherwise. None of that is magic. It's training. Same rules as the body: clear intent, small reps, patient practice.

Mental strength is often sold as hardness—white-knuckle your way through and win by out-suffering others. That's not strength; that's noise. Real strength is awareness plus choice. You notice what your mind is doing, you decide what you'll do next, and you carry on. You don't need to feel brave to act like a competitor. You need a plan for what you'll do when you don't.

Confidence, the kind that lasts longer than a good split, is built from evidence. Not big heroic evidence—stacked small wins. You train when the weather sulks. You stop a rep early because your form is going, not because your pride is. You rewrite a session mid-run so the quality survives the day. You do a hundred of those and something changes: doubt still visits, but it stops making decisions.

Clarity → action → evidence → belief → repeat. It's a loop, not a lightning strike.

Laura arrived on the other side of injury with a head full of warnings. Every niggle meant doom, every hard breath meant she'd lost it, every missed session was a character flaw. She didn't need a harsher plan. She needed proof she could train without lighting herself on fire. We gave her simple mental reps. A one-word focus for each session—flow, steady, light—so she had something to aim her attention at. Two minutes of breathing before key workouts—long exhales, slow starts—to teach her system calm on purpose. Short visualisations twice a week—five minutes, eyes closed, rehearsing the feel of the first kilometre and the awkward middle, not just the finish. A two-line post-session note: what showed up; what she chose. By month two she wasn't fearless. She was steady. "I don't panic anymore," she said. "I reset." That's mental performance. It doesn't always look like fire. Most days it looks like not leaving.

You don't need to overhaul your personality to train your head. You do need to make mindset as visible in your week as intervals and long runs. The simplest way is to build a mental warm-up, a mid-session rescue plan, and a short cool-down for your brain.

Mental warm-up: two minutes, always the same. Stand or sit. Inhale through your nose; exhale longer than you inhale. On each exhale, drop your shoulders. Then speak the session purpose out loud in one sentence: "Today is controlled hard." "Today is easy on purpose." Finish with one cue you'll actually hear later—five words or fewer—because long speeches evaporate at race effort. That's it. You've told your nervous system what day it is.

Mid-session rescue: three steps when you wobble. Step one, name what's happening without the story—"pace drift," "breath tight," "legs loud." Step two, change one thing for two minutes—lift cadence, relax hands, lengthen exhale, sip now. Step three, decide at the end of those two minutes—carry on, scale, or stop. That's how you avoid negotiating for fifteen minutes while your session dissolves. You gave yourself a process; now you follow it.

Cool-down for your brain: write two lines. One on feel, one on choice. "Faded at rep four; slowed cadence, finished cleaner." This isn't a diary. It's a record of what you did when it mattered. In four weeks you'll see a pattern. Patterns are where confidence lives.

Cues are part of the toolkit, but they need to be yours. Short, boring, repeatable. The aim is direction, not inspiration. Before a start: Nerves mean I care. Early in a threshold set: Strong legs, calm head. Mid-race wobble: You've been here; you finish. When thoughts spiral: Let it pass. Stay here. Late push: Posture. Cadence. Proud. Try them in training. Keep the ones you actually hear. Retire the ones that feel like theatre.

Visualisation earns its place when you make it specific. Two or three times a week, five minutes. See the course you'll meet, or a local stand-in. Start with the boring parts: the walk to the start, the first minute of running on tired legs, the second buoy when people clatter. Let your heart rate rise in your imagination and practise calming it: long exhale, cue words, small choices. Rehearse one obstacle each time—dropped bottle, watch freeze, stitch—and rehearse your response. The goal isn't a highlight reel. It's familiarity. On race day your brain will recognise the scene and spend less energy translating.

There are myths worth binning. "You just have to want it more" confuses desire with capacity. Everyone wants it. The difference maker is the person who built the habits that show up under pressure. "Mental toughness means pushing through everything" turns denial into a virtue. Sometimes the bravest call is to back off or stop. That's not quitting. That's protecting the season. Real toughness is doing the useful thing when it's not the glamorous thing.

Another myth: if you're good, you won't feel nerves. Nerves are a body saying, "This matters." We don't delete that. We channel it. Pre-race butterflies are energy. Give them a job: breathe them out slowly; point them at your first cue; let them ride with you for the first five minutes while you keep the promise you made to yourself about pacing.

Pressure makes people choose badly when they try to outrun it. Better to practise it. You can do that inside normal training. Once a week, add a small pressure rep. It might be the last interval where you ask for even pacing without looking at the watch. It might be a brick where you run the first kilometre calm even when your legs feel like fireworks. It might be a long swim with one "fast-to-calm" section where you spike effort for twenty strokes then deliberately settle. The rep is not about speed. It's about keeping your head attached to your body when the sensations change.

You can also rehearse chaos. In a swim, practise getting bumped and returning to rhythm. On the bike, rehearse a bottle fumble without turning the day into a skit. On the run, rehearse a stitch and the fix—long exhale on the opposite foot for a minute, posture tall, back to work. The race won't surprise you with everything. It doesn't need to. It only needs one surprise you've seen before to feel manageable.

Identity and mindset are the same conversation said two ways. If you act like an athlete when it's tidy but turn into someone else when it's messy, your identity needs reps, not your legs. Keep one sentence you can say at the door—I'm an athlete; I start small and build—and one sentence you can say when a session wobbles—Scale, don't scrap. You don't have to feel like the kind of athlete who says those things. You become that athlete by saying them and then doing what they suggest.

The other identity piece is reset speed. Not fewer slips—faster returns. The athlete with long arcs still misses sessions, still has bad days. They just come back sooner because they don't spend three days telling a story about it. Reset speed is a skill. When you notice you've drifted, shrink the ask: a short easy session today; a proper sleep tonight; one quality rep tomorrow. You're back. No ceremony required.

It helps to know your mental red flags. They tend to be predictable. Maybe you catastrophise early—one slow split and the entire day is ruined. Maybe you bargain—I'll push this one rep and quit if it still hurts—and then you keep quitting. Maybe you compare—every training partner becomes a judge. Write the one that catches you most often. Write the counter-move you'll use next time. Catastrophising? "One split is weather; three splits is a trend." Bargaining? "Decide after two minutes of calm." Comparing? "Run my line."

And if your mind loves numbers so much it drowns you, constrain them. One metric per session you actively watch. Heart rate on an easy day. Power on a steady bike. Lap pace on threshold. Let your notes handle the rest. You can't chase five signals at once without turning focus into static.

Because mental work feels abstract until you give it a shape, here's a compact routine you can start this week.

Before key sessions: two minutes breathing (exhale longer than inhale), say the purpose, choose one cue. During: if wobble, name–change one thing for two minutes–decide. After: two lines—feel, choice. Twice a week: five-minute visualisation of a tricky part of your race or a session. Once a week: write a confidence ledger—five quick ticks, not paragraphs—sessions started on time; nights you slept like it mattered; times you adapted without scrapping; moments you fuelled before you faded; one decision you're proud of that won't show on Strava. That ledger isn't motivational fluff. It's evidence. When taper nerves arrive, you'll be holding receipts.

On rest days, give attention somewhere that isn't performance. Read something that isn't about training. See a person who isn't timing you. The brain isn't a battery you constantly drain and then top up with coffee. It's a muscle that benefits from context. Life outside the plan doesn't dilute the plan. It makes it liveable.

There will be days when the best mental skill is permission. Permission to back off. Permission to fail cleanly rather than thrash. Permission to stop a rep because form is gone and ego wants a souvenir. The athlete who can grant that permission to themselves stays around long enough to become who they were trying to be with all that forcing.

There will also be days when the best mental skill is choosing to go again. Not because you're in the mood, but because the session is the kind that builds you. Those are the days when you stand up, put your kit on, and tell yourself the first five minutes are all you need to decide. Most of the time, five minutes is enough to pull you into the flow. Sometimes it isn't. On those days you end early and call it a win for the week. That's judgment. That's maturity. That's how seasons last.

If you want a simple script for race morning, here's one that's saved a lot of athletes from their own heads. Wake up, breathe slow for sixty seconds. Eat what you've practised. Pack what you laid out yesterday. When nerves flare, say this means I care. At the start line, choose two cues—one for form, one for patience. The first five minutes are for rhythm, not proof. If panic arrives, make your world small: breath, feet, the next landmark. If confidence arrives, don't cash it all at once. In the middle, keep your promises—intake on time, decisions steady. At the end, express what's left. After, walk, eat, write two lines. You're not a passenger in your own day. You're the person who makes the small, good choices.

If you only keep a handful of lines from this chapter, keep these. Mindset isn't magic. It's a skill—reps, not revelations. The athlete who resets fastest recovers strongest. Don't wait for race day to think like a competitor; build that voice on Tuesdays. Keep cues short, keep notes honest, keep permission within reach. Train your head the way you train your legs: clear purpose, patient practice, small wins that stack.

Pause & apply: choose one cue for your next hard session, and practise saying it before you start. Add two minutes of breathing to your warm-up. Write the mid-session rescue steps on a sticky note where you can see them. Start a five-line confidence ledger this week. None of this is dramatic. That's why it works.

Chapter 14 – Training with a Life: Chaos-Proof Systems for Real Athletes

Let's be blunt. Most plans weren't written with your life in mind. They were written for a fictional person who sleeps eight and a half hours, eats pre-cut fruit, has a boss who says "Take all the time you need," and trains at the same time, every time, forever. That person does not exist. You do. You have a school run, a late train, a leaking boiler, a partner on shifts, a toddler who thinks 4:37 a.m. is morning. You also have ambitions that deserve better than a plan that snaps the first time Tuesday misbehaves.

So we stop pretending your life is the problem. We make it the blueprint. This chapter is about building performance that fits your world—not squeezing your world into a spreadsheet.

The shift that unlocks everything is small and stubborn: stop chasing the perfect week; chase the consistent month. Perfect weeks are rare. Consistent months are where bodies change and confidence settles. When you hold that frame, missed Wednesdays stop feeling like a verdict. They start feeling like life—absorbed by design rather than derailing the whole thing.

Consistency is rhythm, not rigidity. Rhythm means you know which sessions matter most, which ones can move, and how to shrink or swap without guilt. Rigidity means you tip your week into a bin because one meeting ran long.

Coach's note: the plan that survives your worst week is the plan you'll actually follow on your best.

Here's how we build a week that doesn't snap. First, we choose anchors—the two or three sessions that define progress in your current phase. In a run block, that might be a Tuesday threshold and a Saturday long run. In a tri block, perhaps a Thursday sweet-spot bike and a Sunday long brick. Anchors are the sessions you defend when life swings. Everything else is garnish: useful, nice to have, movable.

Then we create flex, not fiction. One or two sessions exist as "floaters." They have a home, but not a fixed address. They slide forward or back without ceremony. You don't "miss" them if they land elsewhere. You moved them. Language matters.

We add swap logic—pre-decisions you make while calm so you aren't negotiating while stressed. If work explodes, a threshold becomes thirty to forty minutes easy. If the pool closes, you do ten minutes of band work and shoulder shapes before a short spin. If your legs are wooden but your head needs rhythm, you walk tall for twenty minutes and call it training on purpose. You don't need to call it anything else.

And finally, the recovery override: sleep and stress get a vote. If you're two nights short on sleep, quality drops off the calendar unless you truly cannot move it. If you're ill below the neck, you rest. If life is loud enough that you're running on fumes, you halve the ask and keep the habit. The body hears the gesture.

None of that makes you soft. It makes you durable.

Max thought he couldn't follow a plan because he worked hospital nights. The rota changed weekly. Some weeks he felt like a ghost at midday; others like a vampire at 2 a.m. He had three attempts at "proper training" behind him and three quiet collapses to show for it. We didn't give him motivation. He had that. We gave him a frame.

Three anchors, one per sport. A Sunday evening check-in where he looked at the rota and we dropped the pieces into the gaps that actually existed. A red-flag list he could spot with tired eyes: two short nights in a row, appetite gone thin, easy sessions trending faster all week because anxiety wore a cape that said "work ethic." When the red flags stacked, the week simplified—no threshold, just rhythm. His compliance didn't go to 100%. His clarity did. Training stuck. Progress followed. Not because he found extra hours, but because he stopped pretending the old hours were ever coming back.

Planning around real life looks less like a manifesto and more like five practical questions you answer before the week begins:

When are your most reliable time slots? Early morning before the house wakes? A lunch hour on Tuesdays and Thursdays? Saturday early before football? Put anchors there. Don't be heroic; be honest.

Where do you always lose energy? Friday night? Post-bedtime? The hour after your commute? Stop placing quality there and calling it discipline. You're not lazy. You're designing for reality.

Which sessions drain you and which sessions return you to your life calmer? Some athletes' long run is therapy. Others need the swim to quiet their heads. Give yourself the one that helps you be a better human on the hard days.

What does a minimum viable week look like? Write it. One quality, one long, one technique or strength. If everything burns, defend those and let the rest float. A minimum viable week repeated beats a "perfect" plan abandoned.

What will you do when you miss? Not if—when. Pre-write the rule. "I don't cram. I carry on scaled." Future-you will thank past-you for the mercy and the instruction.

Travel, school holidays, work spikes, grief, joy—these are not interruptions. They're the environment training lives in. The mistake is to treat them all the same. The fix is to match the week to the trigger.

Travel weeks are for anchors plus movement snacks. Pack bands, not guilt. If there's a bike, it's a bonus. If there's a pool, it's a gift. Stairs, walks, strength shapes, short runs near the hotel while the kettle boils—that's enough. Choose a view rather than a watch. Your season doesn't hinge on doing sweet-spot in a stairwell.

When kids are off school, you lower volume on paper and raise patience at home. You trade a long session for two shorter ones wrapped around family time. You bring them to the track for relay games while you do strides. You remember that consistency across a decade beats mileage across a week.

When work peaks, threshold leaves the calendar unless sleep stays respectable. You lean into low-cognitive-load sessions: Z2 rides, easy runs, swims with one cue. You put the fast hat back on when your head has space again. Grit isn't doing everything at once. Grit is doing the right thing when it costs you pride.

When your brain is fried and your chest is tight and your body is physically fine, that's not "soft." That's nervous system overload. You regulate first: breathe, walk, light movement outdoors, talk to a human who isn't asking you to perform. Hard will still be there tomorrow. Your job is to still be here too.

Systems make this easier because they reduce decisions when you're most decision-poor. You don't need a new personality. You need fewer frictions.

Stage your kit the night before, even if you "might" train. The presence of shoes by the door moves a morning from 0% to 60% before your brain gets a vote. Load bottles after dinner. Save warm-ups as favourites so you don't think. Pair a session with a habit you already have: bands while the coffee brews; mobility while the pasta boils; ten minutes of shoulder work when you open the laptop for the first time. The point isn't productivity. It's momentum.

Use anchor language at home. Not "I have to train," which sounds like a burden for everyone. Try: "Tuesday night is my threshold hour; Saturday early is my long ride; Thursday I'm home for bedtime." Clarity invites cooperation. Vagueness invites conflict.

Share the calendar with the people who share your life. Not the whole plan—just the anchors, and what you'll protect for them in return. "I've got Saturday 7–9 a.m.; you have Sunday 9–11." The domestic logistics are part of the training plan. Smooth them and the sessions go up in quality without touching your VO2 max.

Coach's note: if your plan requires secret training, the plan is broken.

We use "If–Then" rules to pre-solve chaos without turning you into a robot. If I sleep under six and a half hours two nights in a row, then quality becomes easy and I defend bedtime. If my easy heart rate drifts ten beats high on a cool day, then I slow down or stop, hydrate, and try again tomorrow. If I miss two sessions, then I do a minimum viable week and don't cram. If a niggle speaks twice in the same place, then I change one variable the third time— surface, shoe, duration—and I don't argue.

These rules aren't there to make you delicate. They're there to make you durable. The athlete who makes fewer heroic decisions makes more finish lines.

Not all hours are equal. Learn your chronotype and live kindly inside it. If you are the rare bird who loves 5 a.m., protect evenings for sleep like you protect your bike. If you're an evening engine, stop trying to turn yourself into a sunrise saint because a podcast said so. Put anchors where your energy actually lives. The goal isn't to win mornings. It's to train.

For most people, the pre-work slot is reliable and the lunch slot is a decent second choice. The post-work slot is volatile. It belongs to other people's emergencies and your own fatigue. If you must use it, keep the ask small: technique, strides, mobility, easy Z2 spin. Try not to put your whole season on a slot your boss controls.

Minimum effective weeks carry confidence because they give you a way to "win" when life plays rough. Write a version for 3, 5, and 7 available hours.

If you only have three hours, you still get better: one quality hour (threshold or sweet-spot), one long hour (steady with calm), one mixed hour (technique swim or strength plus a short easy run). If you have five, you add a second sport touch and a brick jog. If you have seven, you lengthen the long and keep one session playful. At every tier, frequency beats heroics. The plan stops being something you fall off. It becomes a ladder with rungs you can actually reach.

On months where you're coasting across a rough patch—new baby, new job, new stress—you can live at three hours without turning into a cautionary tale. On months where life breathes, you climb to five or seven without pretending you'll hold it forever. That's grown-up training. It's less sexy and more repeatable.

Let's walk a chaotic week, because examples stick. You plan a neat block: Tuesday threshold run, Thursday SS bike, Saturday long ride with a brick. Monday night the boiler dies. Tuesday you text the plumber and your session evaporates. In a rigid plan, you panic, move the run to Wednesday, keep Thursday as is, then try to run long Saturday and discover your legs have left your body.

In a chaos-proof plan, you defend the week's job, not the week's order. Tuesday becomes twenty minutes easy at dinner time, purely to keep the habit thread and bleed stress. Wednesday becomes your threshold, but scaled—three reps instead of four, even if you "feel fine." Thursday stays easy; you don't stack two quality days just because a calendar says "Thursday." Saturday you ride long as planned and keep the brick short, because you're clever on purpose. You finish the week feeling like an athlete rather than a person who keeps breaking promises to themselves.

That feeling is the point. It's the difference between showing up next week and quietly drifting.

You can steal time without stealing from yourself. Ten-minute mobility stacks add up. A five-minute breath session before bed is worth more than a doom-scroll and leaves you better for tomorrow. A micro-set of strength (two rounds of hinge, split squat, row, carry) before a run turns joints into allies. You're not "doing more." You're doing smarter.

The same principle holds with food. Put fuel in places that go missing: a bar in your work bag, a bottle on your desk, a banana next to your keys. Decide post-session meals before you start the session so fatigue doesn't choose. Eat when you're busy precisely because you're busy. Under-fuelled chaos feels like lack of discipline. It's biology with a marketing budget.

Sleep gets two lines, because you'll want to skip this and it matters more than you wish it did. Two defended nights a week will carry you further than any supplement. Put them on the calendar, even if the "defence" is just turning your phone off at 9:30 and leaving the kitchen less tidy than you like. Being a little behind on dishes hurts no one. Being a lot behind on sleep hurts everything.

Social training can be a gift or a trap. Keep one session each week for friends and fun. Let the others serve the plan. If your long run always becomes a brawl because your mate can't count to Zone 2, either shorten it, start earlier, or be the boring one who says "I'm staying easy." Boring wins marathons. Drama wins brunch.

If you're the person who invites everyone and then resents the pace, choose solitude for your anchors and people for your floats. Your training doesn't need to be a community project to be valid. It needs to be yours.

Because you'll ask for scripts, here are three that de-escalate life in two sentences or less.

With family: "My anchor this week is Saturday 7–9. I'll be back for breakfast and the food shop. When do you want your slot?" It's amazing how often this turns into a plan rather than a negotiation.

With work: "I'm offline 7–8 on Tue/Thu. If something's truly urgent, call—otherwise I'm back at eight." Most emergencies survive an hour. Your anchors might not survive a culture of instant replies.

With yourself: "If I start and it's clearly not the day, I do twenty minutes easy and stop proud." Permission in advance removes theatre later.

None of this means you never push. It means you push when the ground will hold you. When life is calm, add a rep. When sleep is golden, edge the long ride. When your head is spacious, try the hill session you've been avoiding. When you're tired, don't audition for a resilience documentary. Get home with something left. That's how seasons last.

You'll still have weeks that go sideways. You'll still miss sessions. You'll still sit on the edge of your bed wondering whether you're serious enough to stand up. Serious isn't the sprint to the door. Serious is the system that makes standing up probable most days and graceful to skip when it isn't.

If you only keep a few lines from this chapter, keep these. Training should support your life, not compete with it. Consistency doesn't mean every day; it means enough, over time. Your plan isn't fragile if it's flexible. Anchors define progress. Flex absorbs chaos. Swaps protect momentum. Recovery isn't a mood; it's a rule. The athlete who plans for mess wins more tidy days.

Pause & apply. Tonight, pick your two anchors for the next seven days and put them where your energy lives. Choose one float session and label it "moveable." Write one If–Then rule you'll actually follow. Stage your kit. Put a bottle where you'll see it. Tell one person your anchor times and give them theirs. Then go to bed on purpose. That's a chaos-proof plan. It doesn't look heroic. It looks repeatable.

You're not a robot. You're a human doing something remarkable—fitting training into a full, complex, brilliant life. When you stop fighting your schedule and start building with it, the week feels lighter, your sessions land cleaner, and the month starts to look like progress on purpose. That's the whole game.

Chapter 15 – Nutrition That Fuels

Fuel that works in real life (with expert insight from Rachel Trott, Level 3 Diet & Nutrition Coach)

Before we talk carbs and kitchens, credit where it's due: the backbone of this chapter comes from Rachel Trott, our in-house nutrition coach at Smart Performance Coaching. Rachel's superpower is making food practical. No fads. No fear. Just fuel that fits a real week and supports real training.

You don't need a new personality to eat well. You don't need a scale on the counter or a spreadsheet on the table. You need a few clear ideas you can trust, used often enough that your body knows what's coming. The aim here is neat: eat in a way that lets you train, recover, and live without turning meals into homework.

The simplest way to think about fuelling is in windows. The rest of your eating can stay gloriously normal. Three windows cover most of what matters: before you train, during longer efforts, and straight after. That's it.

Everything else is breakfast, lunch, dinner, and something that tastes good at 3 p.m.

Before you train you give your body what it will ask for later. That means carbohydrate for available energy and a little protein if the gap since your last meal is long. Think porridge with banana; toast with eggs; yoghurt with oats and berries; a smoothie with fruit and oats; rice cakes with nut butter if the clock is rude. If your stomach is touchy at dawn, keep it small: half a banana and a few sips of milk; a couple of chews; a small yoghurt. You're not trying to create a banquet. You're trying to avoid asking your body to run a session on fumes.

During is only for the longer stuff—roughly past the seventy-five to ninety-minute mark for most, sooner if the intensity is honest or the heat is high. Carbohydrate arrives in small, regular parcels: little sips of a drink, half a bar, a gel every twenty to thirty minutes. Electrolytes matter more than people like to admit, especially sodium. You don't need to become a chemist; you do need to use a product you tolerate and a schedule you can remember.

After, within the next hour and a half, you replace what you used and you repair what you stressed. Carbs to top up stores. Protein in the region of twenty to forty grams to support muscle repair (size matters here—the smaller you are, the lower end still works). Real food beats powders when life allows; powders are a tool, not a personality. Eggs on toast, rice and chicken, beans on a baked potato, a sandwich and fruit, yoghurt and granola, chocolate milk if you've got nothing else in reach. No drama. Just something.

Outside those windows? Eat like a human trying to feel good and train well: regular meals, colour on the plate, protein spread through the day, carbs matched to the work, fats that help food taste like food.

Ben is the neat story here. He kept "bonking" on long runs and decided he had a character flaw. He'd roll out of bed, sip some water, and hope. Ninety minutes later he'd be counting lampposts and bargaining with himself. We changed almost nothing about his plan and everything about his fuelling. Toast and nut butter before he left. A gel every thirty minutes once he hit the hour mark. Chocolate milk and oats when he got home. The wall didn't disappear because he got brave. It disappeared because his brain and muscles had a supply line.

He didn't need a new training plan. He needed more food at the right times.

Rachel's first principle is boring and powerful: carbs are fuel, not a moral debate. If your training load is up, your carb demand is up. Your legs don't care about internet arguments. They care about glucose. On heavier days, you lift the carbohydrate content of your meals and snacks. On recovery days, you let it drift down a notch because demand is lower. You're not "good" or "bad." You're matching the work.

Second: protein is repair. A simple target most endurance athletes tolerate well is around 1.6–2.0 grams per kilogram of bodyweight per day, spread across meals and snacks— not dumped into one dinner. Think a palm-sized serving at each meal and a little in snacks. Yoghurt, eggs, dairy, lean meats and fish, tofu, tempeh, beans, lentils, protein-rich grains—choose what you eat happily. You're not trying to become a lifter. You're trying to give your body the building blocks it uses to adapt.

Third: fat isn't the villain and it isn't the hero. It's part of a meal that keeps you full and makes food taste like something you look forward to. Use a sane amount and don't let it crowd your plate off the days you need carbohydrate to show up early in a session. If you're fuelling a pre-run meal, keep fat and fibre modest so the stomach clears in time; put the olive oil elsewhere.

Fourth: hydration is energy in disguise. Dehydration by even a small margin feels like poor fitness. Most of the time it isn't; it's a dry brain and thick blood. Drink water across the day, add electrolytes on long or hot sessions, and don't wait until your mouth is dry. The bottle on your desk is not decoration.

Fifth: there are no "good" or "bad" days in the kitchen. There are days you ate more; days you ate less; days you ate late; days you ate out. Food isn't a morality tale. If last night was chips in the car after training, fine—what's the plan this morning? Guilt and secrecy are poor coaches. Curiosity and adjustment are better ones.

Tracking has its place. For some, a few weeks of logging intake teaches portions, highlights gaps (often protein), and shows where calories were leaking. Then you graduate. If logging makes you anxious, if you're skipping social meals to protect your numbers, if you're panicking over a missed macro—stop. You learned what you needed. Now use structure and feel.

Structure is simple: build meals around protein, colour, and carbs. If you're training hard, the carb portion grows. If you're not, it shrinks. Feel is hunger as data, not a threat. If appetite vanishes when you increase load, that's a nudge to liquid calories or softer foods after sessions. If appetite roars in the evening because you under-fuelled all day, that's a nudge to eat earlier and stop blaming the 9 p.m. snack for a 9 a.m. problem.

A few practical pieces clean up most kitchens:

Breakfast that behaves: if you train early, have a small pre-session bite and a proper breakfast after. If you train later, make breakfast a real meal—oats with fruit and yoghurt; eggs and toast with tomatoes; a bagel with cheese and ham; beans on toast with a side of fruit.

Lunch that lasts: protein plus carbs plus colour—leftover rice and salmon with salad, wrap with chicken/beans and veg, soup with bread and cheese, hummus and roasted veg with couscous.

Dinner that digs you out: don't shrink this meal out of habit if you trained. Pasta with meatballs or lentils; stir-fry with rice; curry with naan; chilli and tortillas; baked potato with beans and cheese. If you don't fancy heavy food, go softer—risotto, noodle bowls, soups with bread.

Snacks that aren't theatre: yoghurt and fruit; a banana and peanut butter; crackers and cheese; trail mix; a small smoothie; chocolate milk; a flapjack on big days. You're not trying to impress anyone. You're trying not to arrive at training empty.

If you live with others, eat with them. You can meet your needs inside normal food. You're an athlete, not a separate species.

On the bike, intake is a skill. You practise it. Start early, sip often, and use the terrain. Tailwinds and flats are for chewing and sipping; headwinds and climbs are for pedalling. On the run, plan for simpler textures—gels, chews, or drinks—because bouncing is a thing. If your stomach complains, it's usually three culprits: too much too late, not enough fluid with your carbs, or a gut that hasn't been trained. Solve for those before deciding you're "sensitive."

Gut training is exactly what it sounds like. You practise the race intake inside training, gradually increasing what you take on across weeks until your body says "this is normal." You don't attempt 60 grams of carbs per hour out of the blue and then write a memoir about how it didn't suit you. You start at 30–40, you see how it goes, you step up. You also practise drinking. Carbohydrate needs water to leave the stomach comfortably. Long sips beat big gulps.

Electrolytes aren't a marketing scheme; they're a tool. Sodium matters for fluid balance. If you're a heavy, salty sweater, you'll often need more than the default tabs supply—especially on the bike in heat. You don't need precise lab numbers to improve. You need a product you like the taste of and a plan you stick to.

Caffeine is optional and useful. If your stomach tolerates it, a moderate dose before a race or late in a long session can help you feel less like a lampshade. The key word is moderate. If coffee turns you into a tambourine, skip it.

Race week eating is grown-up boring. You don't reinvent your diet. You shift portions. Across the last forty-eight hours you let carbohydrate nudge up—extra bread, rice, pasta, potatoes, fruit juice if you like—so stores are topped up. You don't turn every meal into a challenge. You keep fibre and fat moderate the day before if your gut is lively, and you choose familiar foods over experiments. Salt your food a touch more if the day will be hot. Drink normally; don't drown. If you're travelling, take known snacks with you and stop relying on the hotel shop as your performance plan.

Race morning is a copy of something you've done. Eat early enough that you aren't rushing and simple enough that the food leaves your stomach before the gun. If nerves are real, drink some calories. If you can't face a bowl, face a bar. You aren't trying to prove that you love porridge. You're fuelling a job.

"Body composition" is the phrase that derails more seasons than a missed long run. It matters in the sense that carrying strength and less unnecessary mass often makes moving easier. It matters less than people worshipping the scale think it does. Performance improves fastest when you train consistently, fuel the work, and sleep. If you're under-fuelled, you don't adapt; you also raise your risk of illness and injury. If your menstrual cycle disappears or changes for reasons unrelated to contraception, that's a red flag for low energy availability—raise intake and speak to someone qualified. If you're constantly cold, always sore, and weirdly proud of being hungry, that's not discipline. That's trouble dressed as virtue.

If you do choose to change body composition, choose a calm part of the year, not a peak. Adjust slowly. Keep protein high. Keep strength in. Keep carbs around key sessions. Stop if performance dives. You're not chasing a look. You're supporting a craft.

Vegetarian or vegan athletes can meet every performance need with planning. Protein sources shift—beans, lentils, tofu, tempeh, seitan, soy yoghurt, dairy if you include it—and variety earns its place. B12 if you're plant-only, iron awareness for everyone who tends to run low (especially menstruating athletes), and calcium plus vitamin D if sunlight and dairy are light on the ground. None of that is a crisis. It's a shopping list.

If you've had gut issues forever, keep a short log: what, when, and the session. Patterns appear. Sometimes the fix is as simple as spreading fibre more evenly, moving garlic and chilli to meals not within three hours of running, or adding a bit more fluid with your carbs. Sometimes it's worth seeing a specialist. Spend effort where it pays you back.

Travel weeks are for pragmatists. You don't diet in airports. You choose the best option you can. Add protein where it's missing. Carry snacks that save you from vending machines. Ask for an extra banana at breakfast and pocket it. Drink water like it's your job. If you're in a culture with glorious food, eat it. Performance is not asceticism. One excellent dinner won't derail the season. A week of under-eating because you're nervous might.

Family weeks and holidays: fuel enough to train, and train the amount that lets you be there. That is not a compromise. That is the point.

Because the internet loves certainty, here are a few "usuallys" that are safe to keep.

Usually, the reason your evening hunger feels like a monster is because you under-fuelled breakfast and lunch. Eat earlier, and the monster shrinks. Usually, the reason your easy run felt like concrete is hydration and sleep, not a failing personality. Drink and go to bed. Usually, the reason last gel sat like a brick is that you left it too late and tried to cram. Start earlier, sip smaller, carry on. Usually, the reason your weight leapt two kilos on Monday is salt and glycogen, not destiny. Stop fighting water. Usually, the reason your mood is bleak at 9 p.m. is because you haven't eaten enough for the day you did. Have a snack and brush your teeth.

Coach's note: fewer narratives, more meals.

You can make this chapter practical in five minutes. Tonight, sketch tomorrow's fuel around your session. If you're training in the morning, place a small pre-session bite by the kettle and a real breakfast in your calendar. If you're training at lunch, take a snack at 10:30 and plan lunch at 1:30, not 3. If you're training after work, eat a proper afternoon snack so dinner isn't a raid. Fill a bottle now. Put it where you'll see it. If your long session is at the weekend, buy your fuels with the food shop, not at the petrol station.

If you live with people, tell them the simple plan: "I'm eating early on Tuesday because of training; Wednesday's dinner is normal; Saturday I'll eat when I get back and then I'm all yours." You don't need everyone to become your nutritionist. You need them not to be surprised.

If you only keep a few lines from Rachel's playbook, keep these. Food is fuel, not a test. Your body needs carbs. Your ego doesn't. Protein repairs; spread it out. Hydration pretends to be fitness; fix it before you blame your legs. Use tracking to learn, then stop when it starts to own you. Eat more on big days and less on quiet ones. Practise race intake in training. No meal redeems you. No meal ruins you.

Pause & apply: pick the window you neglect most—before, during, or after—and upgrade it this week. If you always start long sessions empty, lay out a simple pre-fuel tonight. If you under-eat during, buy what you'll use and set reminders. If you forget recovery, put a protein-plus-carb option on your shopping list and make it automatic. Two minor changes done often beat one heroic overhaul you abandon.

Food isn't the enemy. It's your rocket fuel, your recovery kit, your consistency. When you learn to eat for performance and sanity, training stops feeling like a fight and starts feeling like a rhythm you can live inside. Next up: how to coach yourself like a pro—thinking clearly about your data without letting it run the show.

Chapter 16 - The SPC Race Strategy Playbook

You've trained. You've tapered. You've eaten like an adult with a plan. Race morning arrives and the loudest question isn't "am I fit?"—it's "will I execute?". That's what this chapter is for: a calm, clear way to turn fitness into a day you're proud of. Not a guess. Not a drama. A blueprint.

Racing well is rarely about suffering more. It's about making smarter decisions earlier, then defending them when the noise turns up. The tools are simple: a pacing plan that starts conservative and finishes honest; a fuelling plan you've rehearsed; a small bank of cues you can hear at high effort; and a backup plan you actually use when something goes sideways. Know your numbers. Know your mindset. Know what you'll do when the race doesn't care about either.

Race week doesn't need to feel like superstition. Think of it as a gentle descent, not a cliff. You keep frequency, trim volume, touch race intensity in short, tidy bites, and go to bed a little earlier than your ego suggests. Two or three days out you confirm logistics: start time, bag drop, travel, where the toilets are, what the course does when it gets bored. The day before you lay your kit out, you stick your fuel where your hands will be, and you stop scrolling forecast threads as if refreshing will change the wind.

A good race week has one page of clarity: when you'll move, what you'll eat, what you'll pack, where you'll stand, and the three sentences you'll use when your head gets loud. That's it. Not bravado. Instructions.

Warm-up is not a ritual to appease the gods; it's how you tell your body what game you're about to play. If you're racing short and sharp—5K, 10K, sprint tri—arrive with enough time to actually warm up. Ten to fifteen minutes easy, a few drills if you use them, four to six short pickups that rise toward race cadence, then a short calm before the start. If you're racing long—half marathon upwards, Olympic tri or beyond—keep the warm-up modest. You're going to warm up in the first miles anyway. Five to ten easy, a couple of strides to remind your brain what legs do, then keep your powder dry. In the water, "fast-to-calm" is the whole show: twenty strong strokes to find space, then you deliberately settle. You are rehearsing the first minute you will meet.

The last thing you do before the gun is breathe out slowly. Not for magic. For signal. Long exhale, shoulders down, one sentence: First five minutes are for rhythm, not proof.

Pacing is where most good days go missing. The start line is designed to make you brave and stupid at the same time; your job is to be neither. You don't "bank time." You borrow from a loan shark who collects with interest at halfway. The fastest versions of you start controlled, settle into honest work, and save expression for the end.

On a 5K, the first kilometre is a test of restraint. Ease five to ten seconds slower than goal pace, feel your shoulders drop, then slide to target and hold. At four kilometres you ask for more posture, more cadence, and you spend what's there without flailing. On a 10K, the first two kilometres are a little boring by design, kilometres three to seven are steady and stubborn, and you lift attention—not heroics— at eight and nine before you run the last one like someone who trained for this. In a half marathon, the first five kilometres are a conversation, not an argument. The middle ten are your job. The final five are posture plus patience plus small additions. In a marathon, the first ten feel like theft; you will want to cash that feeling. Don't. Even effort, quiet fuelling, and a refusal to audition for a documentary are your friends until thirty-five kilometres, where you start counting to landmarks you made up yesterday.

On a triathlon bike, the first ten minutes exist to get your heart rate back under control, get food into the system, and check that your brain can still steer. No surges. The middle is the plan: race-like power or effort, even pressure over terrain, fuelling on the clock. The final ten to fifteen minutes ease one notch—not coasting, just enough to let your run start like you didn't fight a dragon. Off the bike, the first kilometre is quiet feet and a long exhale. Then you go to work.

If you need numbers, use them. If you don't, use feel. What you don't use is adrenaline as a coach.

Fuelling is the other half of pacing. It isn't complicated. It is specific. Eat what you practised, when you practised it. Short races often need nothing more than a decent breakfast and maybe a sip of water on the way. Once you cross the sixty-to-ninety-minute line, the rule is small, regular, and early. Carbohydrate in manageable sips and bites; fluid little and often; electrolytes when heat or sweat rates ask for them. The mistake is waiting until you "need" it. You always "need" it five minutes too late. Build a schedule and stick to it. If the course or crowd breaks the schedule, restart it at the next sensible moment and carry on.

Post-race is still part of race day. Carbs and protein within an hour because your body is soft clay then and you can shape tomorrow's legs as much as you shape today's bragging rights. Salt because you spent it. Water because you're not made of stone. Later you can have the thing you promised yourself at kilometre thirty-two.

Transitions are part of the race, not a tourism break. Walk the route before you start. Find your rack. Count racks from a landmark. Know which side you'll exit. Lay your kit in the order you'll use it. In T1, it's a sequence: unzip, cap and goggles either off and into the suit sleeve or off and in your hand, suit to your waist as you move, then at the bike it's peel, step, peel, step. Helmet on—chin strap first, then touch the bike. That order matters. In T2, it's dismount with room, rack, helmet off, shoes on, grab-and-go with cap and glasses. If you've practised elastic laces, this will feel boring. Boring is fast.

The point of bricks in training wasn't to make you tired. It was to make this feeling familiar. When your legs feel like furniture for the first five hundred metres, smile. You bought that feeling in training so it doesn't scare you now.

The mental part is simple because it has to be. You will not remember a paragraph at threshold. You will remember five words. Keep a small cue bank and use it at set times.

At the start: Breathe, settle, rhythm. At race effort: Strong legs, calm head. When you wobble: Let it pass. Stay here. In the last stretch: Posture. Cadence. Proud.

You're not trying to hypnotise yourself. You're aiming your attention away from panic and towards useful action. Visualisation earns its place if you make it ordinary rather than cinematic. See the queue for the toilets, the shuffle to the start, the messy first minute, the moment the course bites you. Rehearse your response: long exhale, adjust cadence, take the gel, shorten the step, carry on. That way race day feels like déjà vu, not a trial.

There will be chaos. Plan for it now so you don't invent on the fly. Heat will arrive on the one day you packed black. Wind will arrive from the edge of the map. Your watch will freeze. Your stomach will vote against democracy. None of that has to end your day. You need an index card of if–then decisions.

If it's hot, then effort replaces pace and fuelling brings more fluid and sodium; ice or water goes down the jersey; the goal becomes execution under conditions, not martyrdom. If it's windy, then posture gets tall and hands stay calm; you stop surging to prove a point into headwinds and you keep pedalling downhill with light pressure to make the most of tailwinds. If the watch fails, then you race by feel and landmarks: breaths per step, a mantra, the person in front of you reeling in slowly. If your gut turns, then you slow briefly, breathe long, reduce concentration of what you're taking, add water, and give it ten minutes. If you cramp, then you manage position and cadence while you increase intake; if it persists, you adjust your goal to finishing clean rather than collecting a cautionary tale. If you miss a bottle or a gel station, then you take the next available and you don't sprint to "fix it". The race is long. Your body is a forgiving machine if you stop panicking.

Mechanical on the bike? Decide today: quick fix or day over. If you can safely resolve a dropped chain or a simple flat, you do. If you can't, you step aside and live to race properly. Glory doesn't live in trench repairs. It lives in finishing what you trained for most of the time and walking away when it's not your day.

Drafting rules exist and they apply to you. Know the legal distance and the time you have to complete a pass. Ride your plan. Don't build a penalty into your pacing model because you didn't read the briefing.

Marcus is the example of what a one-page plan can do. He's a thinker. On race week he turned into ten thousand tabs. We took him to one page. Top left was warm-up: times, easy minutes, strides, breath. Top right was pacing:

first five minutes conservative, settle to target, cues by kilometre. Bottom left was fuel: what, when, how much, written like a shopping list with times not vibes. Bottom right was chaos: if watch dies, if heat rises, if gut protests. He didn't need a perfect day. He needed fewer choices. He raced like the person he was in training—calm, deliberate, quietly tough.

You can build your own one-pager in ten minutes. Name, bib, start time. Purpose in one line: Express the work with control. Then four small boxes.

Warm-up: what you'll do and when you'll start it. Pacing: first segment conservative, middle steady, finish expressive—define those with either numbers you trust or descriptions you actually feel. Fuel: first intake time, schedule thereafter, what's on the course and what's on you. Cues & chaos: three phrases you'll use; three if–then decisions you'll follow.

Print it. Put it with your kit. Read it once before you sleep and once when you pin your number.

Race morning looks like this. Wake when you planned. Breathe for sixty seconds. Eat what you practised. Sip a little. Leave earlier than you think. At the venue, you move enough to feel human, you queue before you need to, you check your numbers, you lay your things where your hands expect them, and you smile at someone so your brain remembers you like people. When nerves flare, you name them and use them: this matters, that's all. Five minutes before your start, you bring your world small—shoes, breath, first cue. You don't preview the middle. You don't audition the end. You start the first five minutes the way you promised yourself you would.

The middle is always the day. That's where you keep your promises. Intake on time. Effort honest. Posture when you're tired. You use your cues on a schedule, not just when you're in trouble—every kilometre marker, every fifteen minutes, every landmark. You don't negotiate when you're at your worst; you implement what you wrote when you were calm.

The end is your reward. You've earned the right to spend. You keep form tall and feet quick and eyes soft. You run through rather than to the line. Afterwards, you walk, eat, and write two lines you won't forget: one thing you did well, one thing you'll change.

There's a temptation to make every race a referendum on who you are. It isn't. It's a snapshot. Race day is where you express your work, not where you become worthy of it. The smartest strategy is rarely sexy. It's calm, it's clear, and it's been tested enough times that your body and brain recognise it under pressure.

If you only keep a handful of sentences from this chapter, keep these. Start conservative. Hold honest. Finish expressive. Fuel early and on time. Use short cues, often. Plan your chaos while you're calm. When it gets hard—and it will—return to rhythm before you return to pace. You don't have to be fearless. You have to be ready.

Pause and apply. Tonight, write your one-page plan for the next race or hard session. One line of purpose. A first-five-minutes script. The numbers or feels you trust. A fuelling schedule in times, not hopes. Three cues. Three if—then lines. Pack your kit. Put your bottle by the door. Go to bed like it matters.

Race day doesn't change who you are. It reveals what you've practised. With a clear plan and a steady head, you'll race like the athlete you already are.

Chapter 17 - Injury, Niggles & the Smart Comeback

If you train long enough, something will complain. A calf that tightens halfway up the hill. A knee that grumbles after long runs. A shoulder that suddenly remembers you own paddles. This isn't failure. It's training. The question is never "will I get a niggle?" It's "what will I do next?"

This chapter is your comeback guide. Not a miracle fix— not promises that a stretch you saw on the internet will cure all ills. A clear, calm process for spotting trouble early, pausing the right things, keeping the rest of your engine alive, and returning to full training with more confidence than you had before. Comebacks are physical, yes—but they're also mental and emotional. The plan needs to hold all three.

There's no ego in comeback season. Only strategy.

You can think of small injuries like smoke alarms. Some chirp once and stop. Some go off every time you make toast. Some scream because there's a fire. Your job is to tell which is which and act with the right level of urgency.

What most athletes do instead is test the alarm every day: a "just checking" run that teaches the problem to stick around. We're not doing that. We're going to make one good decision, then another, then another, until running (or riding, or swimming) feels like you again.

A straightforward way to start is with a niggle scale:

Green: normal post-session muscle soreness, stiffness that eases fully in a warm-up, background tightness that doesn't change your movement. Train as planned, watch it, add a little care.

Yellow: localised discomfort that lingers, joint stiffness on waking, pain that shows in certain ranges or after a specific duration, tiny spikes that make you think about your gait. Modify and monitor.

Red: sharp pain, swelling, heat, bruising, pins-and-needles or numbness, pain that increases with use, or anything that changes how you move. Stop the trigger, switch the session, decide next steps when you're calm.

Rule of thumb: if pain alters your movement, that's a red flag. Training with altered movement teaches a worse pattern. We want you back fast. That means no rehearsals of a limp.

When something flares, four steps keep you out of the ditch:

Stop the cycle. Don't retest it daily "to see if it's better." Pain is not a riddle you solve by guessing more often. Park the trigger for at least forty-eight to seventy-two hours while you do the rest of the plan around it.

Remove the trigger. You don't have to stop training; you have to stop doing the thing that irritates it. Swap the run for a bike, the bike for a swim, paddles for buoy, hills for flat, lunge pattern for hinge pattern. You're staying an athlete while you fix a part.

Rebuild support. That means calm range of motion, tissue tolerance (strength), and circulation. Light mobility in pain-free ranges, isometrics if appropriate (the "hold" strength that often calms tendons), then progressive loading across days. Movement is medicine—the right kind, in the right dose.

Address the cause. Load spiked? Shoes ancient? Mechanics slipping when you fatigue? Sleep in the bin? Stress turned up? Don't just pat the symptom. Fix the pattern that invited it.

This is not medical advice; it's training process. If your symptoms are severe or you're unsure, see a qualified clinician. Early clarity beats late frustration.

Nina's Achilles is the athlete story that belongs here. Textbook tightness every time she nudged volume. She foam-rolled like it paid rent, felt better for a day, then right back where she started. We stepped off the hamster wheel. No running for three weeks. Calf raises every other day— straight knee and bent knee, slow down, smooth up, within comfort. Hip extension and glute strength work. Ankle range—calm, regular. Walks. Then a walk–run progression that started boring and stayed sensible. She didn't just "heal." She rebuilt capacity. Twelve weeks later she was running faster at the same effort and the ankles were quiet. Injury didn't ruin her progress. It refined it.

The comeback has phases. They overlap, and you move forward when the current one feels too easy:

Capacity first. Keep your engine on. If you can ride pain-free, ride. If you can swim pain-free, swim—with sensible mechanics. If neither is happy, elliptical, deep-water run, or simply walk with intent. Strength circuits that avoid the trigger keep you feeling like an athlete rather than a patient.

Controlled exposure. Reintroduce the pattern that hurt in small, predictable doses. Walk–run is the classic for lower-limb issues: a few minutes walk, a minute easy jog, repeat for fifteen to twenty minutes. If the session is pain-free during and after, and you feel normal the next morning, add a little. If symptoms climb during or after, you either hold or step back. Upper-body issues follow the same logic: range, then light load, then longer levers, then return to sport-specific stress.

Return to structure. Easy volume comes back first. Technique work returns. Threshold comes back last. Long sessions grow on a schedule, not because you feel heroic today. Brick runs stay short and polite until the body proves it remembers how to transition cleanly.

Rewire confidence. This is as important as anything you do in the gym. Most injuries leave a fear: the sharp moment, the step that did it, the hill you've avoided since. We name the fear, write the smallest version of it, do that version well, and then build. Confidence is exposure + success, repeated.

Patience beats bravado. Every time.

Here's what not to do:

"I'll rest ten days and pick up where I left off." You've given the tissue a break, not the capacity to handle the old load. The second climb through volume is when many people tear what they first only irritated.

"I'll run through until I can't." That's not tough; that's how niggles become seasons.

"It's probably nothing; I'll do my long run anyway." Famous last words. If you wouldn't advise your training partner to do it, don't choose it.

Instead, practise this sentence: Scale, don't scrap. And its twin: Resume, don't cram. Those two choices build long careers.

A few common patterns and the simple corrections that save months:

Achilles or calf grumbles: often a load spike, a lot of hills, or shoes that lost their life. Reduce hills for a fortnight, return to flats with short walk–run if needed, calf raise progression, glute work, and slower reintroduction of faster running. Keep strides short and snappy rather than long and jumpy. Check you're not always landing in front of you when tired.

Knee ache (runner's knee feel): look up the chain—hips and glutes; look down the chain—ankle mobility and foot strength. Flatten steep descents for a while. Cadence up five to ten steps per minute can lower joint stress. Strength: split squats, step-downs, hip airplanes, controlled single-leg work, all in pain-free ranges.

Hamstring tugs: often stride length outpacing capacity or power on fast days. Shorten the fast stuff for a few weeks, add hinge strength (RDLs, hip thrusts), and sprinkle isometrics. Don't stretch into pain; build strength through range you own.

Shin niggles: footwear age + sudden volume + hard surfaces. Rotate shoes, reduce impact temporarily, short frequent runs instead of a weekly epic, foot and calf capacity up.

Shoulder for swimmers: heavy paddles + poor scapular control. Ditch heavy paddles, return to buoy + light paddles only if tolerated, scapular Y–T–W, serratus work, and catch mechanics at easy intensities. Breathe out in the water; tension lives in your neck.

Low back on the bike: position plus load. Shorten intervals, lift stack a touch for a fortnight, hinge and anti-rotation strength, and aim for smooth steady pressure rather than spikes.

These are patterns, not diagnoses. When in doubt—or when pain persists—get eyes on it from a pro.

Speaking of pros, red flags that warrant medical assessment:

Night pain that wakes you.

Unexplained swelling, heat, or fever.

Numbness, tingling, or weakness that changes how a limb works.

Pain after a specific pop or snap.

Bone tenderness after a spike in load (think tibia or foot).

Pain that worsens across a week despite rest and modification.

You don't get extra points for ignoring those.

The mental piece is the bit most plans forget. Injury often steals two things: identity and trust. You stop calling yourself an athlete and you stop trusting your body. We fix both with structure.

Identity: you're still an athlete when you walk–run. You're still an athlete when you do band work at the pool instead of laps. You prove that by showing up for the version of training that's available. Keep the ledger going—five quick ticks a week for the choices you made: sessions started on time, sleep defended twice, scaled without sulking, fuelled before you faded, one decision you're proud of.

Trust: comes from doing what you said you'd do and feeling the outcome you hoped for. Write micro-targets you can hit: "today: 6 × 1 min easy jogs that feel boring." Hit them. Next time, add one. You're teaching your brain that your body is not a trap.

Fear in the moment: use a rescue plan. When a sensation appears, name it ("tight, not sharp"). Adjust one parameter for two minutes (cadence up, stride down, effort down). Reassess. If it settles, proceed scaled. If it doesn't, stop the trigger and walk home. You didn't lose a day. You won a month.

A practical return-to-run ladder (adapt the idea to ride or swim as needed):

Week 1 (symptoms calm at rest): 20–30 minutes walk most days. Two or three days of strength: calf/hip/foot or hinge/anti-rotation depending on site. Mobility in painless ranges.

Week 2: 20 minutes walk–run: 4 min walk / 1 min jog, repeat. Every other day. Easy cadence, soft feet. If pain-free during/after and next-morning feel is normal, progress.

Week 3: 25–30 minutes walk–run: 3 / 2, then 2 / 3. Twice. One extra day of cross-training. Strength continues.

Week 4: 30 minutes mostly run: 2 / 4 then 1 / 5. Add a few 10–15 s relaxed strides if everything's clean.

Week 5: 30–40 minutes continuous easy run (or split into two 20s). One very gentle progression segment at the end if you're itching (not required). No threshold yet.

Week 6: Reintroduce one short controlled pickup session: e.g., 6 × 60–90 s "comfortably hard" with full recoveries. Long run grows to 45–60 easy.

Each step assumes symptom-free during, symptom-free that evening, symptom-free the morning after. If symptoms speak, step back one rung, not three. You're building a staircase, not jumping a fence.

For cycling, the same pattern with wattage/effort caps and shorter bouts first. For swimming, volume and intensity progress separately—mechanics first, no paddles until joints and tissues are happy, technique cues to keep tension from living in your neck.

Strength stays the scaffolding. Twice a week in base; once in season. More range and control than load. Full foot on the floor, hips level, ribs over pelvis, slow down phases. Hinge (RDL), split squat, step-down, row/pulldown, carry. Ten good reps beat fifteen messy. Stop a rep in the tank.

Sleep is the quiet accelerant. Two defended nights per week do more for healing than a new gadget. Hydration and protein nudge healing without fanfare. If your appetite vanished while volume dropped, you still need enough in the tank to rebuild tissue—don't starve your comeback.

Ethan's story sits next to Nina's. He strained a hamstring playing five-a-side, then tried to outrun the memory by adding more hard cycling, because it didn't hurt on the bike. Three weeks later his back joined the party. We took the spotlight off speed, put hinge strength back in, cleaned his position on the bike, and returned to running with ten-second strides on grass, building to thirty seconds, then one-minute floats. He hated the slowness and loved being uninjured a month later. Sometimes the "slow" way is the only fast way available.

Common comeback traps and the exit for each:

Testing every day: commit to a 72-hour window without the trigger, then retest with a plan, not a whim.

Binary thinking ("I'm injured/I'm fine"): write the middle: the exercises you can do, the sessions you can swap, the metrics you'll track that don't require pain.

Cramming missed sessions: resume where you are, not where the calendar says you "should" be. The calendar isn't your body.

Hiding it: tell someone. Secrecy breeds bad decisions. Loop in your coach or a training partner so they're not surprised when you scale.

Treating rest like punishment: it's a tool. Use it before the body uses it on you.

You'll want numbers. Here are tidy ones you can use without turning your head inside out:

Shoes: track mileage; most die between 500–800 km. Rotate pairs if you run a lot.

Volume: 10–15% increases are fine on average, with a down week every third or fourth. Big rocks first: frequency before distance, distance before intensity.

Sleep: under 6.5 hours for two nights? Quality session downgrades.

Pain: 0–2/10 acceptable and stable during a return session; 3–4/10, hold or reduce; 5+/10, stop the trigger. Pain that lingers or worsens across twenty-four hours is a red flag.

They're guidelines, not laws. They stop you guessing wild.

The aim isn't to avoid every niggle forever; it's to get good at handling them. The athlete who resets cleanly, rebuilds steadily, and protects confidence will always outlast the athlete who wins Tuesday and loses the month. You can start small and still call it progress. You can back off and still call it discipline. You can walk–run and still call yourself a runner.

If you only keep a few lines from this chapter, keep these. Niggles are information, not insults. An adjusted plan is still a smart plan. Scale, don't scrap. Resume, don't cram. If pain changes how you move, stop the trigger and switch tools. Confidence returns by doing small useful things on purpose, often.

Pause & apply: write your If–Then now. If a niggle appears, then I pause the trigger for seventy-two hours, keep two cross-training sessions, add one strength circuit, and retest with a short, boring session I can end early. Choose the first three exercises you'll do if you can't run (or ride, or swim). Put a note in your phone with a walk–run ladder or a spin alternative. Decide who you'll message if you're tempted to be silly. That's a comeback plan you can actually use.

Injury doesn't mean you've failed. It means your body asked for attention. Give it. Train smarter. Come back stronger—because you chose the boring, repeatable decisions that keep you in the game. Next: how to track progress without letting data run the whole show.

Chapter 18 - Track Less, Learn More – Using Data Without Losing the Plot

If you train with a watch, your watch will have opinions. So will your phone, your bike head unit, your sleep app, and the group chat screenshotting their VO2 scores. None of them have to be the boss.

Data can be brilliant. It can guide your effort, show you progress you'd miss, and warn you before fatigue turns into a layoff. It can also turn training into admin—ten dashboards and no idea how your legs feel. This chapter is a reset. We'll keep the numbers that help, drop the ones that drain, and build a straightforward way to use tech that supports your judgement instead of replacing it.

The outcome we want is very specific: you finish the week knowing what you did, how it felt, and what you'll adjust—without needing to negotiate with a readiness score every morning.

Start with a hierarchy. Not all data is equal, and pretending it is will bury you in noise. Put feel at the top. Rate of

Perceived Effort—RPE—is the only metric that travels everywhere, works indoors and out, on hills, in heat, in wind, and under stress. Right under feel sits consistency: did you train often enough to adapt? Next comes sleep because nothing distorts training like being under slept. Then training load—the rough mix of volume and intensity across the week—because that's how we plan stress and recovery. Then heart rate—resting, during, and how fast it settles—useful with context. Then pace or power—excellent when you know what session you're in and what the numbers are meant to represent. Last, composite tech scores—recovery/readiness/fitness-fatigue. They can be helpful summaries. They can also be confident nonsense if the inputs were off.

The further down that list you go, the less authority a number should have over your day. If your watch says you "need 73 hours of recovery" after a comfortable jog because you forgot to pause at the café, smile and move on.

When does data help? When it guides decisions you were already prepared to make. A resting heart rate that's five beats higher than your normal baseline and sleep that was fractured—use that to downgrade a session you were on the fence about. A threshold workout where the same RPE now produces a slightly faster pace or higher power—use that as proof the process is working. A long run where your heart rate drifted steadily upward at the same pace in heat—use it to reinforce that hydration and shade matter rather than to declare yourself unfit.

When does data hurt? When you react to single points as if they were trends, chase numbers instead of executing the session, or ignore context—travel, heat, arguments, deadlines—and let an app call you "ready" when you aren't, or "unrecovered" when you feel fine and the plan says easy anyway.

Use data to guide, not decide. Let effort lead. Let numbers confirm.

Dani is the before-and-after worth remembering. She had everything: HR strap, GPS watch, sleep tracker, HRV app, power metre. Her training wasn't failing; her head was. She spent more time comparing graphs than noticing how she felt. We didn't throw tech away. We simplified. RPE notes after key sessions. A weekly check-in with three one-to-five scores—energy, sleep, motivation—and a line of context. Pace or power tracked closely in two workouts a week; the rest "good enough." Within a month she felt lighter. Within two months training improved. Progress followed because attention returned to where the work happens.

More tracking isn't more progress. The right tracking is.

So, what's "right"? A lightweight weekly loop you'll actually do:

After key sessions, write two lines: one sentence of feel ("legs heavy, breathing okay"), one lesson ("set off too quick; next time first rep shorter").

At week end, spend five minutes: totals for time or distance (to observe, not to chase), a quick scan of training load (did hard days stand out and easy days stay easy?), and those three feel scores—energy, sleep, motivation.

Mark one proof that isn't in the file: ate on time in the long ride; cut a rep to protect form; left the phone outside the bedroom and slept.

That's your data. Everything else is optional.

Let's talk about the numbers athletes misread most.

Heart rate is the most honest liar in your kit. It reflects heat, dehydration, caffeine, stress, altitude, sleep, excitement, and then training. Use it like a thermometer, not a report card. If it's high on an easy day, slow down and call it a win. If it's suppressed and you feel flat, don't force heroics. In threshold work, if HR won't rise despite effort, you might be carrying fatigue; if it jumps and floats, heat or stress may be driving it. In long runs or rides, watch drift— if the same pace/power costs more beats later, decide whether heat/hydration explains it; if not, the load might need trimming.

Pace is honest on the track and a liar on hills, in headwinds, and when pavement temperature is trying to fry eggs. Treat it as a result of the right effort, not a target at all costs. Power responds faster to changes, especially on the bike; it's exceptional for controlling efforts and learning terrain, but it's only as good as your setup and your ability to keep posture when you're tired.

HRV/readiness can be useful if you collect it consistently and treat it as a trend, not a command. A down-trending week after travel? Nudge load down. A red morning after eight hours of solid sleep, no illness, and your plan says "easy 30"? Go for a walk run or spin and reassess after ten minutes. You're not a lab. You're a person.

The most dangerous number is any single number you let define you.

Practical safeguards keep you out of trouble when tech gets loud.

Pre-session intent: write the purpose, the primary control (RPE, pace, power, or HR), and the exit plan if today isn't the day. Purpose shrinks choices. Exit plan removes guilt.

In-session cues: two prompts you'll actually use—"even pressure," "breathe low," "quiet hands," "cadence steady." Cues beat panic.

Post-session notes: those two lines. Without them, your fancy file is a picture with no caption.

That loop will teach you more in six weeks than a new device will in six months.

A word on zones. They're helpful as a shared language. They're harmful when they become law. Your Zone 2 today in heat won't look like last week's on a cool day. Your threshold on a bad night's sleep will feel worse at the same number. Zone systems differ—five-zone, seven-zone, colour-coded—but they're all trying to map effort to physiology. Pick one, define it with the best information you have (field tests, recent workouts, how it actually feels), and accept that it's a sketch, not a courtroom document.

Testing doesn't need to be theatrical. Every four to six weeks, include short field checks inside normal training: a

20–30-minute controlled-hard run with even pacing; a bike set with 2 × 8–12 minutes hard, full recovery, best effort noted; a swim of 400 + 200 with steady pacing. Look for trends that line up with feel. If you had one heroic day or one awful one, don't rewrite zones. Revisit at the next check.

Heat and altitude deserve their own line because they warp numbers fast. In heat, heart rate will be higher at the same power or pace; let it be. Scale the day by RPE and finish cleaner. In altitude, pace sinks while RPE rises; the best early weeks are controlled, not corrective. You can't argue a mountain down. You can decide to run easy and adapt.

Sleep trackers are useful as habit mirrors, not tribunals. If yours says 6.1 hours with fifty-seven minutes of REM, don't go full detective. Ask simple questions: did I go to bed on time? Wake in the night? Drink water? If yes, protect two nights this week; downgrade a quality session if both nights miss. We don't need to dissect sleep architecture to act like adults.

Steps, floors, calories burned—fine if you like them, irrelevant to training decisions. Don't turn recovery days into scavenger hunts.

Data and identity interact. If you tie your worth to a split, you will be dragged by it. If you grade your day by a watch verdict, you'll learn to ignore your instincts. Language helps here. Swap "I have to hit X" for "Today I'll run controlled hard and stop when form slips." Swap "Zone 2 must be Y pace" for "Zone 2 will let me talk in full sentences on the flat; on hills it's my breath that leads." Small language shifts protect big decisions.

You can also write scripts for predictable arguments with your device. If the watch calls your easy run "unproductive," your reply is "easy runs are not for productivity metrics." If your head unit says "recovery 72 hours" after a session that was clearly moderate, your reply is "noted; tomorrow is easy anyway." If your HR strap drops to 35 bpm mid-interval, your reply is "strap slipped; RPE wins."

Coach's note: fewer stories; more decisions.

Group rides and segment culture are data traps disguised as community. Keep one ride for fun. Let the others serve the plan. If you join a fast group the week you aimed for even sweet-spot work, either change the plan upfront or skip the ride. Don't pretend you'll sit on and then chase every sign. That's not discipline; that's self-deception with a headwind.

Strava is a public diary. Use it as a log, not a stage. Write what you did and what you learned. Hide the suffer score. Private notes tell the truth. Public leaderboards tell a story that often isn't yours.

A clean, low-friction setup keeps tracking in its place:

Auto-lap by kilometre/mile on runs so you can review splits without poking at your watch.

Data screens that match the session: for easy days, time + one metric; for intervals, lap pace/power and lap time; for long endurance, time, current effort, and a fuelling reminder field. Less to look at = more to execute.

One platform you actually read. If your files scatter across three apps, pick one to be the source of truth.

Naming convention you'll use: put purpose first ("Run — Threshold 3 × 8" / "Bike — Z2 + 2 × 20 steady"). Future you will thank you.

Notes field as standard: two lines, always.

If you resent your setup, you won't use it. Make it boring and reliable.

How do you know if you're relying on data too much? A few tells: you won't start a run if your watch is at 9% battery; you call sessions "ruined" when GPS is messy; you feel anxious without a strap; you re-interpret a good-feeling day as bad because a readiness score was low; you won't scale a session you're failing because the plan said four reps. The fix isn't to throw tech away. It's to put feel back in charge for a period.

Try a feel-week: keep tech recording in your pocket or on your bars but set the screen to time only. Execute sessions by RPE. After, look at the file and see how your feel mapped to numbers. You'll recalibrate faster than you think. Most athletes come out of a feel-week with more confidence and fewer arguments with their wrists.

Progress markers that matter are a mix of objective and lived. Objectively: a threshold session performed with tighter control; long runs or rides with better fuelling and steadier effort; swim sets with cleaner splits and less panic. Lived: feeling calmer at the same effort; sleeping better; needing fewer pep talks to start; finishing sessions with something in the tank on purpose. Track both. Post one screenshot if you like. Keep the other three wins in your notes.

Red flags in data that deserve action, not anxiety: easy days creeping faster each week because you can't bear the number; threshold sessions turning into rescue missions; a three-to-five beat resting HR climb across a whole week with lower mood and worse sleep; heart rate not rising on hard sessions and you feel dulled; a readiness trend red without obvious cause and your easy pace feels loaded. Action looks like pulling one hard session, protecting two nights, fuelling properly for forty-eight hours, and writing one sentence that starts with "I'm adjusting..." You don't need a summit. You need a lever.

Make the data serve the season. In base, use numbers to protect frequency and keep easy. In build, sharpen in two key sessions a week while letting the rest be boring and clean. In peak, numbers guard against searching—short bites at pace, not tests. On race week, they anchor rehearsals and then get out of the way. On race day, they sit behind feel when conditions shift. After the race, they support reflection without rewriting your identity.

To put this all to work right now, do this:

Tonight, choose three things you'll track every week—and three you'll stop. Keep: session RPE, weekly feel (energy/sleep/motivation), and time/distance totals. Drop: the readiness score's mood swings, obsession over sleep-stage minutes, and segment hunting as validation. Set your device screens to match your next two sessions. Write tomorrow's purpose and exit plan on a sticky note. After the session, write two lines. Repeat for six weeks.

If you only keep a few sentences from this chapter, keep these. Data is useful when it helps you train on purpose. Feel leads; numbers confirm. One number never tells the story. You are not your watch's verdict. Track the right things. Ignore the noise. Train like a human—not a spreadsheet.

Pause & apply: What's the one metric you grip too tightly? Put it on the bench for a week. Use RPE and your two-line notes instead. At week's end, compare outcomes. If training felt lighter and quality held, you just found room to breathe.

Chapter 19 - The Morning Training Myth

Early training has a reputation it didn't ask for. Own the morning. Win the day. Grind while they sleep. It sounds noble until the alarm goes off and the room is cold and your brain is negotiating with your duvet like it's a hostage situation. Morning training isn't glamorous. It's logistics. It's a decision you move earlier in the day so the rest of the day can't take it from you.

You don't need to become a sunrise evangelist. You don't need an identity transplant. You need a routine that works often enough to matter. For many athletes that routine happens to fit best in the morning, not because dawn is magic but because life gets noisy by 9 a.m. This chapter is about building that routine in a way a real person can live with—quiet, practical, repeatable.

Why bother at all? Because mornings simplify choices. You train before inboxes multiply and small problems become large ones. You make one decision—stand up—and the rest follows. There's less talking yourself into it, less room for "I'll go later" to become "I didn't go." It's not that morning sessions are somehow physiologically superior. It's that they're available. Training that exists beats training that lives in the calendar.

There are real barriers. Dark. Cold. Body not awake. Family life moving at a different speed. A job that sometimes asks for late nights. None of those make you a failure. They make you normal. The question isn't "am I a morning person?" The question is "can I set up two or three mornings a week that work often enough to free the rest of the week?" That's the gain: not hero stories—consistency.

The first lever is the night before. Morning training is won at 9:30 p.m., not 6:00 a.m. Kit staged where you step. Shoes untangled. Bottles filled. Watch charged. Head unit synced. Towel waiting. If you swim, bag packed with a spare cap and the goggles that don't leak, not the experimental pair that fog at the fun bit. If you ride indoors, fan ready, programme loaded, towel on the bars. If you run, route chosen and light charged. If breakfast needs prep, prep it. If coffee helps, set the timer. The more you remove friction, the less willpower you need. Friction is what kills 6:00 a.m.

Then set a micro-script for the first five minutes after the alarm. No scrolling, no compare-and-contrast with your past self, no weather debate. You stand up, bathroom, sip, kit on, out or on. If you want a mantra, make it a verb: stand. By the time you've finished the sip, you're already moving.

"Won't I be too tired to perform?" Sometimes. Which is why not every session belongs in the morning. Early in a build, or when life is heavy, move easy volume and technique to morning and keep the big quality where you can give it the best chance—often later in the day. As your body adapts, some quality can live in the morning too, especially bike intervals indoors or threshold runs you've rehearsed. The rule isn't moral—it's practical: morning gets the sessions you can execute well in that state.

Sleep deserves respect here. If early training steals sleep, you'll pay for it. The fix isn't to be tougher; it's to be earlier the night before and gentler on morning intensity until your system catches up. Two defended early bedtimes a week will do more for performance than a third espresso shot and stubbornness. If you're a shift worker, your "morning" is whenever you wake. Don't copy someone's sunrise just because it photographs well.

A body that has been horizontal for seven hours likes a gentle warm-up. Build a five-minute pre-session that wakes patterns without draining them. Runners: cat-camel, ankle circles, a few calf rocks, ten slow bodyweight squats, then start easier than you think and let stride length gradually appear. Cyclists: hip openers, a few standing calf raises, shoulder rolls, then five minutes of very easy cadence before the work. Swimmers: band Y–T–W, scapular push-ups, two slow long exhales to find rhythm, then 200 easy as 25 drill/25 swim. The point isn't to perform circus tricks in your kitchen. It's to turn your systems on, not shock them.

fuelling before dawn can be simple. If the session is under forty-five minutes and easy, a glass of water may be enough if dinner was sensible; add a small banana or a gulp of juice if you're a light eater at night. If the session is longer or has quality, give yourself some carbohydrate—half a bagel with honey, a small bowl of oats, an easy-to-digest drink—nothing heavy, nothing clever. Coffee helps some, hinders others; learn your own response. What you don't do is treat early training like fasting theatre and then wonder why the wheels come off at minute thirty-eight.

There's a psychological trick that helps more than any gadget—the ten-minute rule. You don't commit to the whole session at 5:59 a.m. You commit to starting. Ten minutes in, if you still feel like stopping, you have permission. Almost nobody uses the permission. Momentum is stronger than motivation. The rule works because it bypasses the most fragile part of the morning—the doorway.

Lucy learned this the useful way. She was a steady evening trainer until work crept into evenings and weeks became a collage of "I'll go later." We negotiated two early sessions a week. We kept the first three weeks deliberately boring: easy run with two strides, then coffee; short swim with mechanics, then home; no intervals at dawn until the body trusted the pattern. The first week she hated it, the second she tolerated it, the third she messaged: "It still isn't fun getting up. But it's less bad than missing." Two months later she still calls herself a night owl. She also happens to train most Tuesdays and Thursdays before the city wakes and the rest of her week is calmer because those anchors are done.

What about intensity at dawn? It can work. It just needs more care. Threshold running before breakfast will feel a notch harder. Sweet-spot cycling pre-work can be excellent—indoor control, no traffic, clean execution. Fast pool work is fine once you're warm; sprinting on no food and two hours of sleep is not "tough"—it's a coin flip. If morning is your only slot for quality, scale the first two weeks: slightly shorter reps, a touch more recovery, and cues that emphasise rhythm over bravado. When it's reliable, nudge back to full.

Inside all of this is a simple idea: protect the anchors; let the garnish float. If mornings are where your anchors live, defend them in the calendar. Everything else can move or shrink without guilt. A calm ten minutes before school drop-off beats a mythical sixty you never start.

Safety matters when streets are empty. Lights, high-vis, routes you know, a message to someone if you're going far. Indoor setups prepped so you don't power-drill in slippers. In water, know when lane times actually begin; don't make the first ten minutes a fight for space because you arrived late and feverish.

If early training means family logistics, loop people in. Two mornings a week you're out; two mornings a week you're on breakfast duty. Swap cleanly, not resentfully. A plan everyone knows is lighter to live.

If mornings fail, don't mythologise the failure. Make an If–Then now. If I miss the alarm, then I move the session to lunchtime at reduced volume or twenty minutes after work and call it a bridge, not a coup. If sleep was broken by a kid or a cough, then I walk the dog and swap the harder work to Friday. If I string two missed mornings together, then I schedule one evening on purpose and reset rather than chasing my tail. This is not moral philosophy. It's event management.

Travel weeks and early meetings deserve their own paragraph. The fix is not to give them your immune system. Travel week mornings are "keep the frame" weeks: one short quality you can execute in a hotel gym or on a quiet loop, one longer easy session (walk-run, spin, pool if you can find one), and a lot of mobility. Set a realistic floor—two sessions—and be proud when you hit it. That pride buys momentum when you return.

Some will ask about hormones, circadian rhythms, science. Yes, time of day can shift perception of effort and performance a notch. Many people feel sharper mid-afternoon. Many have a chronotype that dislikes dawn. The lesson isn't "mornings are best" or "afternoons are best." The lesson is "train at the time you can do most consistently and learn the adjustments that make that time work." If mornings are yours, build the routine and accept that early quality asks for more warm-up and better fuel. If evenings are yours, defend the slot and stop pretending the morning myth applies to you. Identity follows what you do most, not what you post about.

A small thing with large effect: end well. Morning sessions should finish with a minute of calm, not a door-slam sprint into emails. Two long exhales, a drink, a note: one sentence of feel, one sentence of lesson. That sixty seconds stitches training into your day as a stabiliser, not a thief. It also trains your brain to file the morning as "good use of time," which makes tomorrow easier to start.

Another small thing: a minimum effective morning. Give yourself a default plan you can do half-asleep and still call the day a win. Ten to twenty minutes. Runners: 3–4 km easy or 10 × 60 s easy, 60 s walk. Cyclists: 20 minutes Z2 with two one-minute spin-ups. Swimmers: 600–1,000 m mechanics into steady. If you do nothing else all week, those keep you connected. When life returns to normal, the bridge is short.

You'll have weeks where morning training feels like a superpower. You'll have weeks where it feels like a prank. The metric isn't how inspired you felt at 5:45. It's whether the system is light enough to repeat. Two to three mornings most weeks will change your season more than one perfect 90-minute sunrise file per month. Consistency beats cinema.

Avoid common traps. Don't upgrade every morning at once. Don't put your longest long run at 4:30 a.m. because a podcast said grit is a vitamin. Don't sacrifice all evening connection to "be disciplined" at dawn and then resent training for stealing your life. Morning training should make life easier. If it makes it narrower, adjust.

A short map to get started:

Pick two mornings you can protect. Not "in theory"—in your real week.

Move an easy session there for the first two weeks. Keep quality where it fits best.

Build the night-before checklist and put it in one place. Stage the kit where your feet land.

Write the ten-minute script and stick it by your alarm: stand, sip, kit, move.

Add the five-minute warm-up.

Fuel lightly when the session asks for it.

Finish with two breaths and two lines.

Week three, if you want, upgrade one morning to controlled work. Week five, review: are you calmer? Are anchors getting done? Is sleep intact at least two nights? If yes, keep going. If no, change the mornings or let them go. Morning training is a tool, not a personality test.

Max's week looked nothing like Lucy's. He worked nights in a hospital. His "morning" was 4 p.m. on a Wednesday and 9 a.m. on a Sunday. He thought he was failing because his calendar didn't look like the internet. We picked three anchors that matched his mornings: one post-shift short bike before sleep (fan, bottle, quiet), one swim on his first wake day (lanes were empty), one long run at the start of his off-block. He stopped fighting an imaginary schedule and started training inside his own. His consistency doubled, not because he became a morning person, but because he found his mornings.

If you only keep a handful of lines from this chapter, keep these. Morning training isn't about being elite. It's about getting to the work before the day gets away. The win isn't a heroic file—it's starting. Sleep matters more than slogans. Two or three simple mornings most weeks will move the needle more than a complicated plan you don't start. Coffee can be a warm-up. So can water. So can standing.

Pause & apply: pick two mornings in the next seven days. Stage tonight. Write the ten-minute script. Choose the minimum effective session so the bar to "win" is low. When the alarm goes, don't decide how you feel about training. Decide to stand. The feeling follows the first step, not the other way around.

Mornings aren't magic. They're quiet. And in that quiet, before the world begins to pull, you can put your training where it can't be taken.

Chapter 20 - Behind the Scenes – How a Coach Thinks

Pull up a chair. This is the bit most athletes never see: the quiet decisions behind your plan, the reasons your long run moved, the recovery week that appears "out of nowhere," the message that says "cut the last rep and finish clean." Coaching looks like workouts on a calendar. It's really pattern-spotting, fatigue-management, translation, and trust. System + experience + empathy + caffeine.

You don't need a coach to train well. But it helps to think like one. This chapter is a tour of the mental model we use at Smart Performance: what we notice, how we decide, when we change course, and why your plan is a living thing. No mystique, no magic—just the craft of keeping a human moving forward in a messy world.

When we start a season, we don't write sessions. We write a story. Where are you now, where are you headed, and what threads will carry us from here to there? We sketch the big pieces first: anchor days that fit your life (the long ride window that actually exists, the Tuesday evening track you can reach, the swim slot that opens after school drop-off). We protect two to three of those anchors and let everything else float. We note constraints without apology: shift work, childcare, a knee with history, a pool that closes on short notice. These aren't obstacles; they're the blueprint.

Then we ask better questions than "what's the plan?" Questions like: what is this athlete ready for this week? What will their recovery look like given their life, not a laboratory? What confidence do they have now, and how do we build it? Which weakness, if improved, gives the largest carryover? If we push here, where do we make space? Every decision sits on top of those questions. The best week on paper is useless if it can't be lived.

From there, we pick a few simple levers to guide the month. Maybe you respond well to frequent touches and struggle with single monster days. Maybe you thrive on structure Monday–Thursday and need deliberate looseness at weekends. Maybe threshold is your friend but Zone 2 creeps fast unless we defend it. We don't drown you in rules; we install rails you can feel.

And then we watch.

A coach reads more than splits. We read language. "Legs heavy, head fine" is different from "head flat, legs okay." "HR high but felt smooth" is different from "couldn't find a gear." We read cadence lines that sag in the last third. We read breathing cues buried in your notes. We read what isn't written—the four days you suddenly stopped logging sleep, the emoji that disappeared, the quiet apology in a message that starts "sorry for letting you down," which really means "I'm losing belief."

Numbers matter. So does the pattern behind them.

Common early signals we act on: a three-to-five beat climb in resting heart rate for a full week, easy efforts feeling "loaded," more caffeine but flatter mood, a drift of easy pace upwards with the same RPE, and a run-on sentence in your notes where you convince yourself to push again tomorrow. We don't wait for a crash. We change something now: pull one hard session, insert a true easy day, defend sleep twice, add carbohydrates for forty-eight hours, write a micro-win you can hit tomorrow. The aim is not to prove you're tough. It's to keep you in the game.

Sometimes our job is to be the brakes. You arrive with ambition and a work ethic that could power a small town. You stack sessions, label it momentum, and kayak straight towards a waterfall. Good coaching keeps the river but steers you away from the drop.

Sometimes our job is to be the gas. You've built base, you're strong, and you still tiptoe into every effort like you need permission. You don't need a hug. You need a clean push: "Today we go." Not redlining for theatre—sharpening because the season asks for it.

Most of the time, our job is quieter. We remove friction. We remind you why this session is small and important. We tell you to end while moving well, not to feed an app. We help you translate the messy week at work into training decisions that don't punish you for being human.

Jamie is the "just tell me what to do" athlete you've met in your club. Capable, drowning in choices. His life ran on deadlines and late calls. He'd open a plan, overthink everything, then train randomly and feel guilty. We simplified:

Fewer sessions, more impact.

Hard early in the week, never late Friday.

A midweek reset baked in: twenty minutes easy or nothing, no debate.

We kept two anchors sacred and let the rest be Lego. He stopped negotiating with himself and started executing. Same engine, different steering.

Coaching isn't controlling a calendar. It's decoding chaos into decisions a person can live with.

What you might not see are the calculations under a plan you think is "just a week." We're tracking load on a rolling basis—some use TSS; some keep a mental ledger of hard days and long sessions. We're spacing intensity across disciplines so your Tuesday track doesn't sit on top of your Wednesday bike over-unders. We're considering indoor vs outdoors: the heat load of a turbo, the neuromuscular bite of strides, the shoulder stress of paddles, the reality that your Thursday pool is carnage and your best technique ask belongs on Monday. We're planning one B-race as a learning day, not a referendum, and we're tapering less than you want because we know sharpening is keeping frequency, reducing volume, and leaving teeth in—short, tidy doses, early enough to freshen.

We are also planning the off-ramps. If work explodes, which session drops without touching the spine of the week? If your kid is home with a fever, how do we salvage rhythm with a ten-minute minimum effective dose that counts? If a niggle speaks, what is the exact swap that keeps confidence while we protect tissue?

Those off-ramps are not pessimism. They're kindness engineered in advance.

We keep lists you never see. Athletes who do better on two quality touches than three. Athletes who only need one long run above ninety minutes to race a half well. Athletes whose minds sharpen with a small amount of speed year-round. Athletes who treat a group ride like a court summons and shouldn't go within a mile of it in peak. Athletes whose sleep is the single biggest performance variable.

We also keep phrases we repeat on purpose. "Scale, don't scrap." "Resume, don't cram." "Finish clean." "Today builds tomorrow." They sound simple because they are. Simple is repeatable under stress.

We look for patterns in your year, not just your week. Where do you always wobble? Week seven in a build? After your first excellent race? The fortnight you call "work audit and I hate everything"? We pre-write the plan to change shape there: downshift volume by a quarter, shrink the long day, keep one taste of intensity, widen recovery, and get you out into daylight. You'll say "It's like you knew." We did, because your life has a rhythm. We train with it.

We also remember the months when you didn't believe you were an athlete. Sometimes the best session we write is an easy one you can finish without feeling like you owe us an explanation.

How do we decide to move a long run? Look at the context you can't see in the file. If your Thursday strength session finally loaded your hinge pattern well and your notes say "back tight but good," we're not stacking a hilly long run on that. If the weather swings to heat and you've underfuelled twice this week, we'll slide the long run to a cooler morning or trim it and focus on fuelling on time. If your HRV dipped all week, your toddler was sick, and your boss sent six calendar invites titled "URGENT," we might keep the long run but remove the progression block and tell you brunch is part of the plan. We are not trying to be clever. We're trying not to be stupid.

And when we drop a recovery week exactly where you think it's "suspicious"? It's because planned recovery beats accidental collapse. You will always feel like you could do more on day one of a down week. That's the right time to take it.

We care about what happens between sessions. You learn how to fuel during the long ride, but you also learn how to sit at your desk without turning your shoulders into earrings. You practice identity when you cut the last rep to protect form. You practice confidence when you start after a bad day and finish with one small win you wrote down. A coach's best compliment isn't "you crushed it." It's "you adjusted like a pro."

We have red flags you should borrow for self-coaching. Three negative notes in a row—adjust now. RPE rising while pace/power falls across a week—adjust now. Sleep dipping below 6.5 hours for two nights—downgrade quality. Repeated apologies for missed sessions—address mindset, not compliance. Avoid turning stress into a character flaw. It's a load management problem with feelings attached.

If you're coaching yourself, think like a coach who cares about you. Build a weekly rhythm that separates hard from hard. Protect two anchors; let the rest float. Write the purpose of each session before you start and an exit plan if it isn't your day. Keep a lightweight review on Sunday: what worked, what didn't, what one lever will change next week—sleep, fuel, spacing, or volume. Track feel (energy, sleep, motivation) alongside numbers. Schedule recovery weeks in ink. Use "if–then" plans for predictable chaos: If travel week, then two anchors and a lot of walking; if early niggle, then pause the trigger for seventy-two hours and keep two cross-training sessions. And be kind in your notes. Your brain reads them later and makes decisions based on the tone you set.

You don't have to be your own drill sergeant. You have to be your own best ally.

A few behind-the-scenes plays we run a lot:

We rename sessions to change behaviour. "Tempo" becomes "controlled hard." "Recovery run" becomes "easy means chat pace." Language directs effort more than you think.

We rehearse race day in parts. Not just bricks and pace, but breath under noise and the "fast-to-calm" switch you'll need in open water. We write cue cards you can hear at race effort, not poetry that makes sense only on the sofa.

We use boredom on purpose. Boring files win races. Even pressure, sensible cadence, on-time fuelling. If you never get praised for a dull, well-executed session, you'll chase drama. We praise dull a lot.

We separate emotion from information: a bad day doesn't make you a bad athlete, and a great day doesn't make you invincible. Hold both lightly and stay with the process.

We adjust before you break. You'll say "I could have done more." Exactly. That's why you'll be ready next week.

Alex messaged at 21:37 the night before his race: "I'm panicking. I don't think I've done enough." We didn't send a paragraph about grit. We pulled receipts: three threshold blocks you nailed last month, two long rides with fuelling on time, the open-water set where you went fast to calm without losing your head. Then we wrote tomorrow's script in three lines and told him to put his phone down. He negative-split the run by feel. Fitness didn't change overnight. Belief did, because we pointed it at evidence.

Marcus, the overthinker, was the opposite problem. He had a plan and fifty what-ifs. We gave him one page with boxes to tick and a line for each phase: warm-up, start, middle, late. He raced the page, not the internet. The plan wasn't magic. It was small enough to use under pressure.

Laura came back from injury not trusting her body. We trained her brain as deliberately as her hamstring. Two-minute reflections, visualisation of the scary moments (the first stride, the turn, the surge), one word per session (steady, light, tall). She stopped trying to prove she was fixed. She practiced being fine. Her fitness improved when her nervous system stopped bracing for bad news.

This is coaching. Not tricking you into heroics. Showing you who you already are, then giving you the next clear thing to do.

We also say no. No to stacking races so close your taper becomes a lifestyle. No to paddles for six weeks after your shoulder whispered. No to "I'll do the long run anyway" when your kid was up all night and you had four coffees for breakfast. Not because we love limits but because boundaries build seasons that last.

We accept your life. We plan around school plays, audits, holidays, grief, joy. Training is not an escape from life; it's a part of it. When life grows, training flexes. When life shrinks, training sharpens. The plan is a conversation, not a contract.

If you peeked inside our heads mid-write, you'd hear a hum:

What's the job of this session?

Where is the recovery that actually recovers?

What keeps confidence intact if today goes sideways?

What's the smallest change with the biggest effect?

What will this look like on a bad Tuesday—not just a perfect Saturday?

That hum never turns off. It's why we move your long run when wind turns biblical and your week already screamed. It's why we'll add a nap to your plan and call it training. It's why we'll ask what you said to yourself when the interval went wrong, not just what the watch said.

We're not trying to be clever. We're trying to be useful.

If you only take a few things from this chapter, take these. Good coaching isn't control; it's collaboration. The plan is a living thing built around you, not around a spreadsheet. Adjustments are care, not correction. The best decisions are small and repeatable under stress. The language you use in your notes changes your season. Boring, clean files on ordinary days make extraordinary race days possible.

Stop. Think. Adapt: what does your coach—or your inner coach—need to support most right now: performance, recovery, mindset, or something else? Write the one lever you'll pull this week to help that happen. Earlier bed twice? One true easy day? Fuel on time in the long one? A message that says "I need a lighter week"? Then do it. That's the conversation working.

Coaching is clarity in a noisy world. It's trust built in small proofs. It's seeing potential before it's proven and holding it steady when the week tries to shake it. It meets you where you are, reflects what you do, connects progress to identity—not just outcomes. The goal isn't only a faster race. It's a stronger mindset, a steadier system, a more resilient human who knows how to keep going.

That's the work. That's the art. And it's why the best coaching sticks long after the finish line.

Final Words

You made it.

Not just to the end of a book, but through months of decisions that didn't always feel glamorous: staging kit the night before, starting when you didn't feel like it, cutting a rep when form slid, fuelling on time, writing two honest lines after sessions when a screenshot would've looked prettier. You've done the quiet work people rarely post about. That matters.

You're my favourite kind of athlete — curious. Curiosity is what kept you reading when a slogan would've been easier. It's what got you out the door when motivation hid behind a long day. It's what turns "maybe" into "I did." Curiosity keeps doors open. Training moves through those doors.

This was never a book about becoming perfect. It's a way to train that fits a real life. It asks for purpose, not theatre. It keeps identity at the centre so your plan doesn't fall apart the first time your calendar does. It teaches you to build confidence from behaviour, not headlines. It gives you a handful of simple levers you can pull under stress: slow down, fuel early, finish clean, sleep twice, reset quickly. None of that requires a lab, a monk's schedule, or a personality transplant. It requires a human who's willing to make sensible choices more often than not.

If there's a thread running through everything you've read, it's this: progress is a loop, not a straight line. You reflect, you reset, you repeat — with a little more clarity each pass. The moments you'll remember won't be a single split or a dramatic graph. They'll be the ordinary mornings you trained before the day took your time, the long rides where you ate on schedule and arrived home steady, the swims where you remembered to exhale and the panic never started, the runs you kept easy when ego wanted a story.

You don't need to hold all of it in your head at once. You only need to hold the next clear thing.

So, before you close the book, make it practical. Not complicated — useful.

Tonight, set the stage. Put your kit where your feet will land. Write the purpose of tomorrow's session on a sticky note and stick it to the kettle. Add one exit plan you'll actually use if today isn't the day. Fill a bottle. Choose one cue you can hear in your head when you're breathing hard. That's enough.

Where to go from here? You've got a whole system to play with, but systems need rhythm. Start small on purpose. Give yourself four weeks with boring goals you can actually hit.

Week one: keep two anchors and let everything else float. One quality session you finish with something left; one long easy session you fuel on time; one strength touch you can repeat. Every key session ends with two lines in your notes — feel and lesson. If sleep is thin, make your win a short start, not a long story.

Week two: keep the frame, nudge the detail. Repeat week one with one small progression — a rep added, a minute extended, or five seconds per kilometre off the threshold block because you can do it cleanly. Eat like an athlete on the long one. Protect one early night. Boring on purpose.

Week three: practise the adjustments you'd usually avoid. If work explodes, defend your anchors and drop the garnish without apology. If a niggle speaks, remove the trigger for seventy-two hours and swap in something you can finish well. Write the decision down. That's you coaching yourself.

Week four: step back a quarter. A lighter week you planned beats a crash you didn't. Keep one small taste of intensity so rhythm stays alive. Sleep twice. Touch strength once. At the end of the week, reflect for five minutes: what worked, what dragged, what lever gives you the biggest return next month? Pick one. Move on.

Keep that monthly rhythm and your season will start to feel like a story you recognise: set-up, development, sharpen, exhale. Not perfect — coherent.

You'll still have wobbles. That's fine. When you do, shrink the task. The fastest way back is the smallest honest effort. Ten minutes. A walk-run in trainers you actually like. A twenty-minute spin with a fan and a bottle. A 600–1,000m swim where your only job is long exhale, quiet hands. Momentum returns because you made it easy to begin, not because you argued yourself into inspiration.

You'll also have weeks you want to chase. If you catch a tailwind — good sleep, good mood, good weather — you don't need to invent heroics. Do the plan well, maybe add one short rep to the session that already asked for it, and bank the feeling. Your body doesn't need fireworks to adapt. It needs repeatable signals, delivered calmly.

Some days you'll hear the old lies. "If I can't do all of it, it's not worth it." "If it didn't hurt, it didn't count." "If the watch wasn't impressed, neither should I be." Those lines aren't facts. They're habits. Replace them with sentences that help: "Small counts." "Controlled hard builds." "The watch is information, not a verdict." Say them out loud if you need to. Language directs behaviour.

A word on identity before you go. You don't become an athlete at the finish line. You become one each time you act like one — often when nobody's watching. It's not a mood. It's a practice. The sentence you wrote earlier in this book still matters: "I'm an athlete who..." Keep it boring and true. For the next month, you are an athlete who trains four times a week, one session can be twenty minutes, easy days are actually easy, and you finish with one in the tank. Build on that. The medal is a by-product.

And a word on community. You become the kind of athlete you see often. Choose people who train like you want to: steady over noisy, kind to themselves with standards, curious about their own process. Share real notes with them once a week — not theatre, not self-loathing. One win, one lesson, one plan. Light accountability beats loud comparison.

If your plan bends under life, remember that it's meant to. Good plans flex early. If your kid is ill, if work throws a week at you, if your body asks for a quieter day — adjust now. "Resume, don't cram" is a sentence worth writing where you'll see it. Cramming is a tax you pay with interest.

Resuming gets you back to consistency faster than guilt ever will.

If you're coming back from a niggle or an injury, take your time and take notes. Remove the trigger, rebuild strength, add exposure carefully, stop a rep early even when you feel fine, and pay attention to the pattern that set it off. Say "I'm rebuilding" rather than "I'm behind." Behind implies a perfect schedule you failed. Rebuilding is accurate — and useful.

If race day is near, keep your plan small enough to use under pressure. Three cues you can hear when your heart's high. A pacing strategy you've practised. A fuelling plan you've already tested. A decision for when it goes sideways: breathe, scale, carry on. You don't need to be fearless. You need to be ready to act like the person who's trained for this.

You may be tempted now to set six goals at once. Don't. Pick one performance goal and one process goal. Maybe it's a race in twelve weeks and a behaviour you'll repeat for eight. The behaviour will carry you when the goal feels far. Add a simple ledger once a week: sessions started on time, nights slept well, times you adapted instead of scrapped, one decision you're proud of that won't appear on a graph.

That ledger grows confidence more reliably than a dozen pep talks.

You might also want to buy things. Gear helps when it reduces friction. It hinders when it becomes a hobby. Choose simplicity that gets used. Tyres with sensible pressures, a watch screen that shows only what you need today, shoes that match your body and your routes, a fan that keeps you honest indoors, a bag that lives by the door. The system is not a catalogue.

Nutrition doesn't need a rebrand every month. Eat enough to support the work, especially carbohydrates around hard sessions. Spread protein across the day. Drink water. Add electrolytes when heat or duration demand it. Save experiments for training, not race week. You'll perform better, and you'll stop wasting headspace where a sandwich would do.

If you coach yourself, keep thinking like a coach who cares about you. Write plans you can live. Schedule down weeks before you feel wrecked. Separate hard from hard. Give every session one job and an exit plan. Ask each Sunday: what worked, what wobbled, what one lever will I pull next week — sleep, spacing, fuel, or volume? Follow your own advice. And use a tone in your notes that you'd use for someone you're trying to help, not someone you're trying to impress or punish.

If you work with a coach, tell the truth. The best adjustments come from honest notes: how it felt, what life is doing to your recovery, where your head is. Coaching isn't control. It's collaboration. When a rest day appears "out of nowhere," it came from somewhere — usually from patterns your coach saw in what you wrote and what you didn't. Trust the calm. Ask questions. Learn the why. Then own it.

You may wonder if this is it — if you're "done" building your system. You aren't, by design. The point isn't to finish learning. It's to keep your system light enough to live with and solid enough to carry you through mess. The structure will evolve. The levers won't. Purpose beats pressure. Identity fuels consistency. Clarity shrinks decisions. Recovery carries load. Simple plans outlive clever ones. Boring files win races.

When you forget (and you will), the headline is waiting:

STOP. THINK. ADAPT.

Stop — create a small gap before you choose. Stopping is not quitting; it's making space to decide. Think — return to purpose, cues, context. What's the job? What will make this a win I can repeat? What's my exit plan? Adapt — scale, swap, proceed, or call it. Finish clean. Log two lines. Move on.

That loop will serve you in training and outside it. It's a way to keep your head when the day, the meeting, the family, the weather, or your watch disagrees with your plans.

Thank you for trusting these pages with your time and attention. You've taken a lot in. You won't remember it all tomorrow. You don't need to. You only need the next clear thing and the nerve to keep it small. Kit by the door. Purpose on the kettle. Two breaths before you start. Ten minutes to win the morning. Fuel before you feel clever. A note after. Early to bed twice. Repeat.

You're built for more than finishing. You're built for growth you can sustain. You're built to run with a rhythm you can hold, to ride with posture you can keep, to swim with breath you can control, to lift with range that keeps you healthy, and to decide with a calm that makes the whole thing possible.

If you get lost, come back here. Or send a message. Or find your coach. Or re-read the chapter that speaks to where you are. There is no shame in resetting. It's a skill. Athletes with long arcs have fast resets. That's not a quote. It's what we see, season after season.

Now close the book. Stage your kit. Write the sticky note. Choose the smallest useful step. Do it. Then do it again on more days than not. That's the work. That's the art. That's how real athletes — people with lives and deadlines and school runs and uneven sleep — build performances that last longer than a finish-line photo.

You've got enough to begin, begin again, and keep going. I can't wait to see what you do next.

Smart Tips Collection

A practical, no-fluff playbook you can use tomorrow morning. Keep the tone simple, the steps small, and the cues short enough to remember mid-effort. Pin this by your turbo, screenshot it for your phone, or print it for your kit bag.

Swim Edition — One Stroke at a Time

Relax your hands. White-knuckle swimming stiffens the whole chain. Imagine holding a crisp, dry leaf between thumb and forefinger—secure, not crushed. Soft hands let the forearm set a cleaner catch and keep the shoulder from hiking. Quick check: Do three strokes with exaggerated relaxed fingers, then close gently and notice how the water "grips" your forearm more than your palm.

Exhale in the water. Most "I can't breathe" problems are CO_2 issues, not oxygen shortages. Slow bubbles out, short inhale in. Don't hoard air. Micro-drill: $4 \times 25m$ "long exhale" (breathe every 3 or 2, but commit to full bubbles) $\rightarrow$ 25m easy swim carrying the same exhale.

Eyes down, neck long. Looking forward lifts the head, sinks the hips. Look down or just ahead of the lane line; imagine a string lengthening the back of your neck. Cue: "Crown long, chin tucked." Test: If you see the far wall more than the black line, your head is high.

Kick from the hips. Tiny, snappy kicks balance the body. Knees bend just enough to flick the toes; think "paintbrush ankles." Mini-set: 6 × 25 kick with snorkel + board held at hips (not straight arms) → focus on hips initiating, ankles loose.

Quiet entry. Fingertips first, hand slides in on the line of the shoulder. Splash is wasted energy. Drill: 6 × 50 as 25 fingertip drag (lightly graze the surface in recovery) + 25 swim feeling the same relaxed recovery and clean entry.

Count strokes—make efficiency visible. Speed lies to you in busy lanes. Stroke count (SPL) tells the truth about drag and length. Set: 6 × 50 building from 2–3 strokes fewer per length than usual, then hold that count for the last two with easy effort. Don't chase pace—chase shape.

Drill with intent, not habit. Two or three drills, done well and then "translated" into normal swimming, beat a bag of toys and random sets.

Scull front (early catch pressure)

6/3/6 (timing + rotation + breath)

Polo/heads-up (posture & sighting) Rule: Always follow drill with swim that carries the same cue for 25–50m. If it doesn't transfer, the drill isn't helping today.

Short, sharp sets. Quality goes first when you're tired. Use 25–100m repeats with short rest to hold form. Example: 3 × (6 × 50 @ 20s rest) #1 easy-steady with cue, #2 controlled hard with cue, #3 easy—repeat.

Practise sighting early. Make sighting boring: every 6–8 strokes, quick chin pop, one goggle out, eyes find the buoy/clock, back to neutral. Pool hack: Place a bottle or pull buoy at the lane end; sight it on schedule for 8–12 × 50.

Finish under fatigue. Race swims start hot and settle; train the "fast-to-calm" switch. Brick idea: 8–10 min easy spin → 6 × 50 (8–10 strong strokes → settle to steady + one sight) → 200 easy. This is race rehearsal in miniature.

Common fixes, fast:

Sinking legs? Press sternum slightly forward, eyes down, small kicks, long exhale.

Crossing over? "Train tracks" hands enter in line with shoulder; feel catch under forearm, not across body.

Shoulder ache? Lose big paddles, shorten repeats, ensure early vertical forearm; add 2 × 8 scapular pulls banded post-swim.

Open water composure checklist:

Suit high in armpits/hips. 2) Three long exhales before start. 3) First minute calmer than you think. 4) Find feet; don't tap them. 5) Two cue words: long exhale / quiet hands.

Bike Edition — Power, Endurance & Focus

Find your cadence range. Most athletes are efficient at 85–95 rpm on flats; climbs tolerate 70–85 if controlled. Cadence too low = grind fatigue; too high = cardio drift. Test set: 3 × 6 min at the same power (low-mid Z3): 75 rpm / 85 rpm / 95 rpm. Note HR and RPE. Keep the one that feels smoothest for steady work.

Pedal smoothly—steady pressure. No stomping. Imagine spreading peanut butter all the way around. Drill: 3 × (2 min single-leg @ easy gear + 3 min both legs smooth). Indoors works best.

Aero you can hold. Fast is "quiet": head still, shoulders soft, hips stable, breath low. If you can't drink, eat, and stay aero, your position's too brave. Cue: "Soft elbows, low breath, quiet head."

Fuel early. Eat before you feel clever. On rides >75–90 min, start carbs in the first 20–30 min; sip fluid every 10–15. Heat demands more. Head unit reminder: lap alert every 15 min—"sip/eat".

Train the way you'll race. Same bottles, same mix, same pockets. Learn what your gut tolerates in training, not at mile 40. Note: what your stomach tolerates indoors doesn't always translate outdoors—test both.

Control the climb. Shift early, sit tall, keep pelvis level; avoid ego surges. Climb set: 4 × 6 min @ Z3 seated, 60–70 rpm, focus on posture → 3 min easy between.

Descend with intent. Eyes through the exit, brake before the turn, light hands, light pedals, slight pressure to keep chain engaged. Parking-lot drill: figure-eights with controlled entry/exit speeds.

Intervals build real-world power. Long rides aren't enough. Two staples:

Sweet-spot: 3 × 12 min @ high Z3/low Z4 (5 easy)

Over/unders: 4 × 6 min (1 min Z4 / 1 min high Z3) (4 easy)

Reframe wind. Headwind = honest resistance; posture + cadence + fuelling. Tailwind = free speed; keep shape, don't sprint every section.

Arrive ready to run. Last 10–15 min: settle HR, fuel, cadence where you want first km of run. Brick cue: "Calm power → calm feet."

Indoor vs outdoor rules: Indoors: big fan, towel, bottles reachable, same calibration each time. Outdoors: route matches the session; out-and-back for even efforts, loops for variety; avoid traffic-light "intervals."

Equipment that matters: Fresh tyres, sensible pressures (follow manufacturer chart), comfy contact points, fit you can hold. Fancy is fun; quiet watts are faster.

Run Edition — Strong Strides (Fresh or Off the Bike)

Cadence check. Most land cleanly at 170–180 spm; the goal is your efficient rhythm. Drill: 4 × 2 min at easy pace: 165 / 170 / 175 / 180 spm. Which feels snappy but relaxed? Keep that for easy days.

Shorten the stride. Overstriding brakes you. Land under your centre of mass; let cadence, not reach, make speed. Cue: "Foot under hip."

Run tall. Ribcage over pelvis, eyes forward, shoulders unshrugged. Test: Final kilometre of easy run—do a 20-second "posture scan": tall–loose–light.

Light landing. Aim midfoot under you. Heavy heel slaps often = overstride or downward reach. Drill: 6 × 20s barefoot strides on grass (or minimal shoes) to teach lightness; walk back recovery.

Brick rhythm matters. Teach the 3–5 minute post-bike wobble. Brick micro-progression (4 weeks):

Wk1: 45–60 min Z2 ride → 8–10 min very easy run.

Wk2: 60–75 min ride with 2 × 10 min steady → 12–15 min easy, last 3 steady.

Wk3: 75–90 min ride with 3 × 10 steady → 15–20 min run building to race feel for 5 min.

Wk4: 90 min ride with 20–30 min race-like block + fuelling → 20 min run (5 easy / 10 controlled / 5 easy).

Effort over pace. Heat, hills, fatigue distort pace. Use RPE and HR guards; protect easy days. Hot-day hack: slow 15–30 s/km at the same RPE, increase fluids, shorten the session if form slips.

Consistency beats perfect. Small, repeatable runs > occasional hero sessions. If time is short, 20 minutes counts.

Drills sharpen economy. Two times per week post-warm-up:

4–6 × 20s strides @ 5K feel, walk back.

2 × 30m A-skips or high-knees, 2 × 30m butt-kicks, 2 × 30m fast feet.

Run tired sometimes, but on purpose. A pre-fatigue run (after Z2 ride) teaches control; keep it short and easy.

Recovery runs are real. If you can't hold a conversation, it's not recovery. Keep it truly easy or walk-run.

Common fixes, fast:

Side stitch? Slow, long exhale; press fingers under rib on the side; reduce jostle for a minute.

Calves scream off the bike? Start with short steps and higher cadence; don't chase pace for the first 5–8 minutes.

Transition Edition — The 4th Discipline

Rehearse T1/T2 until boring. Walk the flow. Swim exit landmarks, rack position, mount line, dismount line. Then practise tired: two bricks before race week with full transitions.

Standardise layout. Helmet front-up, straps open; shoes placed the same way; nutrition staged where you'll grab it. Muscle memory = speed.

Pack minimalist. Only what you use. Every extra object is a decision under stress. Checklist (short course): goggles, cap, suit; helmet, bike, shoes, number/belt; run shoes, cap, gels/sips.

Know your flow. Narrate out loud in practice: "Cap/goggles off into sleeve; zip down; suit to waist by rack; helmet on/strap; unrack; jog to mount."

Small hacks that save minutes: Elastic laces; little talc in run shoes; rubber bands for shoes on bike (if safe and taught); pre-opened gels taped to top tube.

Plan B mentality. Stuck zip? Don't fight; peel from shoulders. Dropped gel? Move on—grab at aid station. Slow buckle? Breathe, try again. Panic is slower than calm.

Mount/dismount practice tired. One session per month: 6–8 repeats rolling mount/dismount at low speed in an empty car park post-ride.

Ease out of T1. Two minutes calm: settle HR, feet flat, breath low, then build. Don't sprint your day away.

Skill, not afterthought. Time your transitions in training once. Review the video if possible.

Top Ten Musts — The Non-Negotiables

Show up, especially when it's inconvenient. Momentum beats mood. Your job is the first five minutes.

Sleep like it's training. Target 7–9 hours when you can; if life won't allow it, bank two early nights a week. Screens out; room cool; routine simple.

Fuel before hungry; hydrate before thirsty. Start carbs in the first half hour on long rides/runs; sip fluid every 10–15 min. Bonks aren't character tests—they're planning errors.

Warm up with intent, not habit. 5–10 minutes that prepare your movement pattern: band Y-T-W for swim; high-cadence spins for bike; mobility/strides for run.

Master basics before chasing complexity. Mechanics → rhythm → load. Fancy sessions don't fix sloppy patterns.

Build your mindset like a muscle. Cues, short visualisations, two-line reflections. Confidence = evidence you can see.

Respect recovery. Schedule down weeks; protect easy days; naps count; walks count; quiet counts.

Own consistency, drop perfect. 20 minutes done now beats 60 mythical minutes later. Scale, don't scrap.

Know your why. Revisit it. Write it where you'll see it on tired days. If your why shifts, let the plan follow.

Act like an athlete daily, not just on race day. Small behaviours—kit staged, bottle filled, exit plan written—create results long before a number pin does.

Quick Reference Cues

Swim — Long exhale. Quiet hands. Hips up. Breathe out in the water, slice the entry, let the legs float behind the line.

Bike — Soft elbows. Even pressure. Fuel early. Relax the upper body, keep power smooth, eat before you feel clever.

Run — Tall–loose–light. Foot under hip. Calm feet. Posture first, shoulders easy, short stride that lands under you.

Brick — Bike calm → run calm. Back off 1–2% late on the bike so cadence and breath transfer clean.

Transition — Breathe. Strap. Go. Exhale once, helmet first, move while you sort the small stuff.

Bad day — Scale, don't scrap. Shorter reps, longer rests, or twenty minutes easy. Keep the thread.

Week view — Two anchors, one flex. Protect two key sessions; let one float wherever life allows.

Always — Finish clean. End with form you'd be proud to repeat tomorrow

Strength — Move well, then load. Full range, stable trunk, one rep in the tank.

Open water — Sight, settle, slide. Two sights, long exhale, stay long between strokes.

Hills — Chest up, quick feet. Shorten stride, drive lightly, don't fight gravity.

Heat — Pace by feel, drink early. Slow a shade, salt + fluids before you fade.

Threshold — Smooth, not heroic. Even splits, quiet breathing, stop one rep early if form goes.

Long run/ride — Start easy, finish tidy. Hold back 20–30 minutes; arrive with form, not drama.

Recovery — Easy means easy. You should be able to chat—and want to keep going.

Sleep — Guard the first hour. Screens down, snack prepped, tomorrow's kit laid out.

Fuel — Carbs on work days. Eat for the session you're doing, not the one you wish you did.

Mindset — Cue, don't argue. Pick one line, repeat it; fewer stories, more decisions.

Tech — One intent, one metric. Hide the rest; feel leads, numbers confirm.

Group day — Smile, stay smart. Share the effort, skip the surges if it breaks your week.

Final Nudge

Don't try to swallow the whole playbook. Change sticks when it's small, obvious, and hard to avoid. For the next two weeks, choose four levers: one swim cue, one bike habit, one run adjustment, and one life rule (sleep or fuel). That's it. Write them where you'll see them: kettle, phone lock screen, turbo, gear drawer. The win isn't finishing a perfect plan; it's repeating a simple one until it feels normal.

Here's how to make it real.

1) Pick what you'll own (not what sounds impressive). Choose the cue you actually need most. If breathing unravels in the water, "Long exhale" beats "stroke count". If you always bonk at 90 minutes, "Fuel early" beats another interval session. If your easy runs creep fast, "Tall–loose–light" beats a new shoe.

2) Write a two-week card. On a sticky note or index card, print four lines:

Swim → Long exhale (every 3rd length, hold form)

Bike → Fuel early (sip every 15 min; carbs start by 00:20)

Run → Foot under hip (cadence steady; no reaching)

Life → Sleep twice before midnight (Tue/Thu)

Stick it where you make coffee. When you forget (you will), the card remembers.

3) Shrink the task before the day starts. Decide your "smallest useful version" in advance. Ten minutes is a session. One gel at minute 20 is fuelling. Two long exhales at each wall is breathwork. A 22:30 lights-out twice per week is sleep training. Tiny is the point—tiny survives chaos.

4) Start without negotiating. You don't need a pep talk. You need momentum. Stand up, kit on, go. Give it ten minutes. If it's not the day, scale and finish clean. If it is, you're already moving.

5) Log two honest lines after key sessions. No essays; just evidence.

Feel: "Legs heavy; breathing calm."

Lesson: "Fuel on time helped last 30 min."

Those lines build confidence faster than screenshots.

6) End the fortnight on purpose. After two weeks, spend five quiet minutes: what worked, what dragged, what one lever gives you the biggest return next fortnight? Keep that, swap one other. Progress is rotation, not overhaul.

What success looks like (it's boring)

You will not feel epic. You will feel steady. You'll notice you started more often, fuelling turned up earlier, breathing stayed calmer, and your notes sound kinder and clearer. That's the goal. Quiet evidence stacks. Loud perfection collapses.

Last word

You don't need to become someone else to do this. You just need a clearer version of you—one who makes fewer decisions, earlier in the day, and lets simple habits carry more weight than moods.

Here's the truth we've circled for a few hundred pages: progress isn't dramatic. It's ordinary decisions repeated with less friction. The long arc is built from short starts. The race-day surge is paid for by quiet weeks where you trained on purpose, ate like an athlete, slept like you meant it, and stopped writing essays in your head about one missed session.

Keep your world small enough to act. Four levers for two weeks. One cue in the water. One habit on the bike. One adjustment in your stride. One life rule you can actually keep. Write them down where your coffee lives. Start before you think about it. Finish before form decays. Leave two honest lines so tomorrow's you doesn't have to guess.

You will have average days. Use them. Average days are where capacity is built because you did the work without theatre. You will have bad days. Cut the session in half, or swap it for twenty easy minutes, or call it. Discipline isn't ignoring signals; it's acting on them quickly. You will also have sharp days. Don't empty the tank every time. Leave a little in your pocket so the next day exists.

Confidence is not a speech; it's a logbook. Stack evidence where you can see it: sessions started on time, fuelling when you said you would, easy days kept easy, a few nights of decent sleep. Read that evidence more often than you read your doubts. The voice in your head answers to what you show it.

If you're stuck, make the target smaller. Ten minutes counts. One drill counts. A gel at minute twenty counts. Laying out your kit counts. These are not consolation prizes. They are the mechanics of momentum. The athlete who learns to begin quickly and scale wisely wins more weeks than the athlete who designs perfect ones and finishes none.

If you're tempted to rewrite everything, resist. Edit, don't overhaul. Keep what worked. Change one thing that didn't. Training that lasts is built like a good paragraph: clear subject, clean verbs, no extra words. Your season should read the same way.

If you want a final checklist, make it this:

Know the job before you start.

Do the smallest useful version immediately.

Stop while you're still moving well.

Write two lines: feel + lesson.

Return tomorrow.

When you forget—and you will—begin again without ceremony. No debts, no speeches. The reset is the skill that keeps you in the game longer than talent or bravado.

You're not chasing a new identity at some future finish line. You're proving it, quietly, in the way you train this week: intent over impulse, structure over drama, patience over panic. Keep the frame. Let the details breathe. And when in doubt, move your body, eat some food, drink some water, and go to bed.

That's it. That's the work. Start small today, and again tomorrow. Let simple wins accumulate until the person who "tries" looks a lot like the athlete who "does."

The SPC Athlete Contract

An agreement I make with myself.

Purpose I'm choosing a way of training that I can keep—one that fits my life, builds confidence, and lasts. By signing, I promise to act like the athlete I'm becoming.

My Promises

Clarity & Intent

I promise to state the purpose of every session before I start.

I will use one intent and one primary metric per session.

I will finish clean—ending before form breaks.

Consistency & Structure

I promise to protect my 2–3 anchor sessions each week.

I will treat other sessions as flex—they can move or be skipped without guilt.

I will write two honest lines after key sessions (Feel + Lesson).

Effort & Pacing

I promise to lead with feel (RPE); numbers will confirm or correct.

I will keep hard days hard and easy days truly easy (no grey-zone drift).

I will scale before I scrap (fewer/shorter reps or longer recoveries).

Recovery & Health

I promise to fuel sessions over 75–90 minutes and eat to recover.

I will respect sleep as training and protect a realistic bedtime.

I will include a deload week (~25–40% easier) every 3–4 weeks.

Safety & Red Flags

I promise to stop or modify if I have fever, chest/GI illness, or pain that changes my movement.

I will act on red flags (rising resting HR, sinking mood, <6.5 h sleep ×2 nights): convert to Z1–Z2 20–40 min or rest, add carbs, sleep early.

I will not cram missed sessions; I'll resume calmly.

Data Sanity

I promise to judge by trends, not blips.

I will let context (sleep, stress, heat, terrain) guide decisions.

I will tidy my screens—only show data I actually use.

Boundaries & Life Fit

I promise to keep training in its place alongside family, work, and health.

I will defend my anchors during busy weeks and let flex sessions go—without guilt.

I will avoid "secret heroics" and "punishment miles."

Consequence & Reward

If I break this contract (ignore red flags / skip deload / cram): I will run a 72-hour reset (Z1 only, fuel, sleep) and then resume scaled.

If I keep this contract for 30 days: I will reward myself with

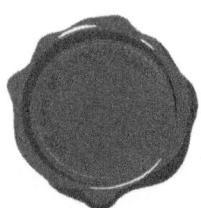

Signature (Athlete):

_____

Date: _____ / _____ / _____